Mometrix
TEST PREPARATION

Oncology Nutrition

Exam Secrets Study Guide

Dear Future Exam Success Story

First of all, **THANK YOU** for purchasing Mometrix study materials!

Second, congratulations! You are one of the few determined test-takers who are committed to doing whatever it takes to excel on your exam. **You have come to the right place.** We developed these study materials with one goal in mind: to deliver you the information you need in a format that's concise and easy to use.

In addition to optimizing your guide for the content of the test, we've outlined our recommended steps for breaking down the preparation process into small, attainable goals so you can make sure you stay on track.

We've also analyzed the entire test-taking process, identifying the most common pitfalls and showing how you can overcome them and be ready for any curveball the test throws you.

Standardized testing is one of the biggest obstacles on your road to success, which only increases the importance of doing well in the high-pressure, high-stakes environment of test day. Your results on this test could have a significant impact on your future, and this guide provides the information and practical advice to help you achieve your full potential on test day.

Your success is our success

We would love to hear from you! If you would like to share the story of your exam success or if you have any questions or comments in regard to our products, please contact us at **800-673-8175** or **support@mometrix.com**.

Thanks again for your business and we wish you continued success!

Sincerely,
The Mometrix Test Preparation Team

Need more help? Check out our flashcards at:
http://MometrixFlashcards.com/Nutrition

Written and edited by the Mometrix Exam Secrets Test Prep Team
Printed in the United States of America

TABLE OF CONTENTS

Introduction

Thank you for purchasing this resource! You have made the choice to prepare yourself for a test that could have a huge impact on your future, and this guide is designed to help you be fully ready for test day. Obviously, it's important to have a solid understanding of the test material, but you also need to be prepared for the unique environment and stressors of the test, so that you can perform to the best of your abilities.

For this purpose, the first section that appears in this guide is the **Secret Keys**. We've devoted countless hours to meticulously researching what works and what doesn't, and we've boiled down our findings to the five most impactful steps you can take to improve your performance on the test. We start at the beginning with study planning and move through the preparation process, all the way to the testing strategies that will help you get the most out of what you know when you're finally sitting in front of the test.

We recommend that you start preparing for your test as far in advance as possible. However, if you've bought this guide as a last-minute study resource and only have a few days before your test, we recommend that you skip over the first two Secret Keys since they address a long-term study plan.

If you struggle with **test anxiety**, we strongly encourage you to check out our recommendations for how you can overcome it. Test anxiety is a formidable foe, but it can be beaten, and we want to make sure you have the tools you need to defeat it.

Secret Key #1 – Plan Big, Study Small

There's a lot riding on your performance. If you want to ace this test, you're going to need to keep your skills sharp and the material fresh in your mind. You need a plan that lets you review everything you need to know while still fitting in your schedule. We'll break this strategy down into three categories.

Information Organization

Start with the information you already have: the official test outline. From this, you can make a complete list of all the concepts you need to cover before the test. Organize these concepts into groups that can be studied together, and create a list of any related vocabulary you need to learn so you can brush up on any difficult terms. You'll want to keep this vocabulary list handy once you actually start studying since you may need to add to it along the way.

Time Management

Once you have your set of study concepts, decide how to spread them out over the time you have left before the test. Break your study plan into small, clear goals so you have a manageable task for each day and know exactly what you're doing. Then just focus on one small step at a time. When you manage your time this way, you don't need to spend hours at a time studying. Studying a small block of content for a short period each day helps you retain information better and avoid stressing over how much you have left to do. You can relax knowing that you have a plan to cover everything in time. In order for this strategy to be effective though, you have to start studying early and stick to your schedule. Avoid the exhaustion and futility that comes from last-minute cramming!

Study Environment

The environment you study in has a big impact on your learning. Studying in a coffee shop, while probably more enjoyable, is not likely to be as fruitful as studying in a quiet room. It's important to keep distractions to a minimum. You're only planning to study for a short block of time, so make the most of it. Don't pause to check your phone or get up to find a snack. It's also important to **avoid multitasking**. Research has consistently shown that multitasking will make your studying dramatically less effective. Your study area should also be comfortable and well-lit so you don't have the distraction of straining your eyes or sitting on an uncomfortable chair.

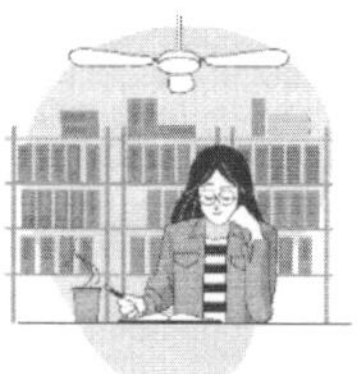

The time of day you study is also important. You want to be rested and alert. Don't wait until just before bedtime. Study when you'll be most likely to comprehend and remember. Even better, if you know what time of day your test will be, set that time aside for study. That way your brain will be used to working on that subject at that specific time and you'll have a better chance of recalling information.

Finally, it can be helpful to team up with others who are studying for the same test. Your actual studying should be done in as isolated an environment as possible, but the work of organizing the information and setting up the study plan can be divided up. In between study sessions, you can discuss with your teammates the concepts that you're all studying and quiz each other on the details. Just be sure that your teammates are as serious about the test as you are. If you find that your study time is being replaced with social time, you might need to find a new team.

Secret Key #2 – Make Your Studying Count

You're devoting a lot of time and effort to preparing for this test, so you want to be absolutely certain it will pay off. This means doing more than just reading the content and hoping you can remember it on test day. It's important to make every minute of study count. There are two main areas you can focus on to make your studying count.

Retention

It doesn't matter how much time you study if you can't remember the material. You need to make sure you are retaining the concepts. To check your retention of the information you're learning, try recalling it at later times with minimal prompting. Try carrying around flashcards and glance at one or two from time to time or ask a friend who's also studying for the test to quiz you.

To enhance your retention, look for ways to put the information into practice so that you can apply it rather than simply recalling it. If you're using the information in practical ways, it will be much easier to remember. Similarly, it helps to solidify a concept in your mind if you're not only reading it to yourself but also explaining it to someone else. Ask a friend to let you teach them about a concept you're a little shaky on (or speak aloud to an imaginary audience if necessary). As you try to summarize, define, give examples, and answer your friend's questions, you'll understand the concepts better and they will stay with you longer. Finally, step back for a big picture view and ask yourself how each piece of information fits with the whole subject. When you link the different concepts together and see them working together as a whole, it's easier to remember the individual components.

Finally, practice showing your work on any multi-step problems, even if you're just studying. Writing out each step you take to solve a problem will help solidify the process in your mind, and you'll be more likely to remember it during the test.

Modality

Modality simply refers to the means or method by which you study. Choosing a study modality that fits your own individual learning style is crucial. No two people learn best in exactly the same way, so it's important to know your strengths and use them to your advantage.

For example, if you learn best by visualization, focus on visualizing a concept in your mind and draw an image or a diagram. Try color-coding your notes, illustrating them, or creating symbols that will trigger your mind to recall a learned concept. If you learn best by hearing or discussing information, find a study partner who learns the same way or read aloud to yourself. Think about how to put the information in your own words. Imagine that you are giving a lecture on the topic and record yourself so you can listen to it later.

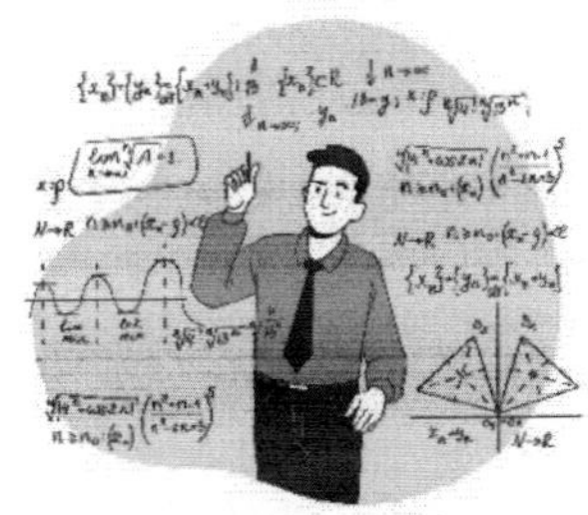

For any learning style, flashcards can be helpful. Organize the information so you can take advantage of spare moments to review. Underline key words or phrases. Use different colors for different categories. Mnemonic devices (such as creating a short list in which every item starts with the same letter) can also help with retention. Find what works best for you and use it to store the information in your mind most effectively and easily.

Secret Key #3 – Practice the Right Way

Your success on test day depends not only on how many hours you put into preparing, but also on whether you prepared the right way. It's good to check along the way to see if your studying is paying off. One of the most effective ways to do this is by taking practice tests to evaluate your progress. Practice tests are useful because they show exactly where you need to improve. Every time you take a practice test, pay special attention to these three groups of questions:

- The questions you got wrong
- The questions you had to guess on, even if you guessed right
- The questions you found difficult or slow to work through

This will show you exactly what your weak areas are, and where you need to devote more study time. Ask yourself why each of these questions gave you trouble. Was it because you didn't understand the material? Was it because you didn't remember the vocabulary? Do you need more repetitions on this type of question to build speed and confidence? Dig into those questions and figure out how you can strengthen your weak areas as you go back to review the material.

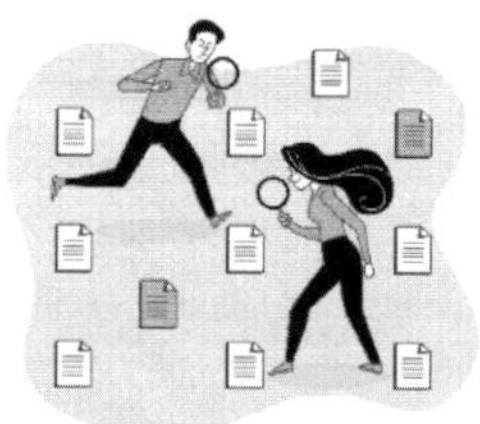

Additionally, many practice tests have a section explaining the answer choices. It can be tempting to read the explanation and think that you now have a good understanding of the concept. However, an explanation likely only covers part of the question's broader context. Even if the explanation makes perfect sense, **go back and investigate** every concept related to the question until you're positive you have a thorough understanding.

As you go along, keep in mind that the practice test is just that: practice. Memorizing these questions and answers will not be very helpful on the actual test because it is unlikely to have any of the same exact questions. If you only know the right answers to the sample questions, you won't be prepared for the real thing. **Study the concepts** until you understand them fully, and then you'll be able to answer any question that shows up on the test.

It's important to wait on the practice tests until you're ready. If you take a test on your first day of study, you may be overwhelmed by the amount of material covered and how much you need to learn. Work up to it gradually.

On test day, you'll need to be prepared for answering questions, managing your time, and using the test-taking strategies you've learned. It's a lot to balance, like a mental marathon that will have a big impact on your future. Like training for a marathon, you'll need to start slowly and work your way up. When test day arrives, you'll be ready.

Start with the strategies you've read in the first two Secret Keys—plan your course and study in the way that works best for you. If you have time, consider using multiple study resources to get different approaches to the same concepts. It can be helpful to see difficult concepts from more than one angle. Then find a good source for practice tests. Many times, the test website will suggest potential study resources or provide sample tests.

Practice Test Strategy

If you're able to find at least three practice tests, we recommend this strategy:

Untimed and Open-Book Practice

Take the first test with no time constraints and with your notes and study guide handy. Take your time and focus on applying the strategies you've learned.

Timed and Open-Book Practice

Take the second practice test open-book as well, but set a timer and practice pacing yourself to finish in time.

Timed and Closed-Book Practice

Take any other practice tests as if it were test day. Set a timer and put away your study materials. Sit at a table or desk in a quiet room, imagine yourself at the testing center, and answer questions as quickly and accurately as possible.

Keep repeating timed and closed-book tests on a regular basis until you run out of practice tests or it's time for the actual test. Your mind will be ready for the schedule and stress of test day, and you'll be able to focus on recalling the material you've learned.

Secret Key #4 – Pace Yourself

Once you're fully prepared for the material on the test, your biggest challenge on test day will be managing your time. Just knowing that the clock is ticking can make you panic even if you have plenty of time left. Work on pacing yourself so you can build confidence against the time constraints of the exam. Pacing is a difficult skill to master, especially in a high-pressure environment, so **practice is vital**.

Set time expectations for your pace based on how much time is available. For example, if a section has 60 questions and the time limit is 30 minutes, you know you have to average 30 seconds or less per question in order to answer them all. Although 30 seconds is the hard limit, set 25 seconds per question as your goal, so you reserve extra time to spend on harder questions. When you budget extra time for the harder questions, you no longer have any reason to stress when those questions take longer to answer.

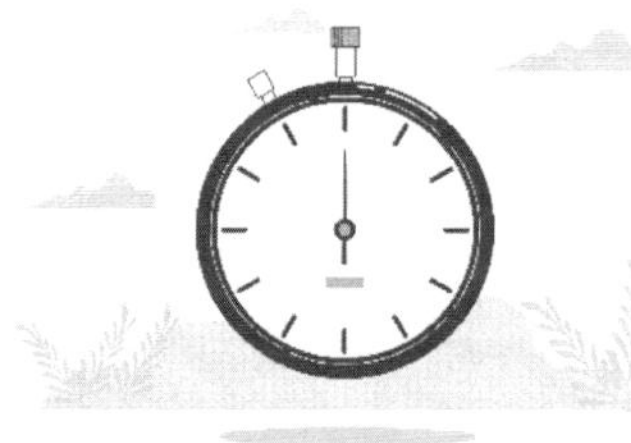

Don't let this time expectation distract you from working through the test at a calm, steady pace, but keep it in mind so you don't spend too much time on any one question. Recognize that taking extra time on one question you don't understand may keep you from answering two that you do understand later in the test. If your time limit for a question is up and you're still not sure of the answer, mark it and move on, and come back to it later if the time and the test format allow. If the testing format doesn't allow you to return to earlier questions, just make an educated guess; then put it out of your mind and move on.

On the easier questions, be careful not to rush. It may seem wise to hurry through them so you have more time for the challenging ones, but it's not worth missing one if you know the concept and just didn't take the time to read the question fully. Work efficiently but make sure you understand the question and have looked at all of the answer choices, since more than one may seem right at first.

Even if you're paying attention to the time, you may find yourself a little behind at some point. You should speed up to get back on track, but do so wisely. Don't panic; just take a few seconds less on each question until you're caught up. Don't guess without thinking, but do look through the answer choices and eliminate any you know are wrong. If you can get down to two choices, it is often worthwhile to guess from those. Once you've chosen an answer, move on and don't dwell on any that you skipped or had to hurry through. If a question was taking too long, chances are it was one of the harder ones, so you weren't as likely to get it right anyway.

On the other hand, if you find yourself getting ahead of schedule, it may be beneficial to slow down a little. The more quickly you work, the more likely you are to make a careless mistake that will affect your score. You've budgeted time for each question, so don't be afraid to spend that time. Practice an efficient but careful pace to get the most out of the time you have.

Secret Key #5 – Have a Plan for Guessing

When you're taking the test, you may find yourself stuck on a question. Some of the answer choices seem better than others, but you don't see the one answer choice that is obviously correct. What do you do?

The scenario described above is very common, yet most test takers have not effectively prepared for it. Developing and practicing a plan for guessing may be one of the single most effective uses of your time as you get ready for the exam.

In developing your plan for guessing, there are three questions to address:

- When should you start the guessing process?
- How should you narrow down the choices?
- Which answer should you choose?

When to Start the Guessing Process

Unless your plan for guessing is to select C every time (which, despite its merits, is not what we recommend), you need to leave yourself enough time to apply your answer elimination strategies. Since you have a limited amount of time for each question, that means that if you're going to give yourself the best shot at guessing correctly, you have to decide quickly whether or not you will guess.

Of course, the best-case scenario is that you don't have to guess at all, so first, see if you can answer the question based on your knowledge of the subject and basic reasoning skills. Focus on the key words in the question and try to jog your memory of related topics. Give yourself a chance to bring the knowledge to mind, but once you realize that you don't have (or you can't access) the knowledge you need to answer the question, it's time to start the guessing process.

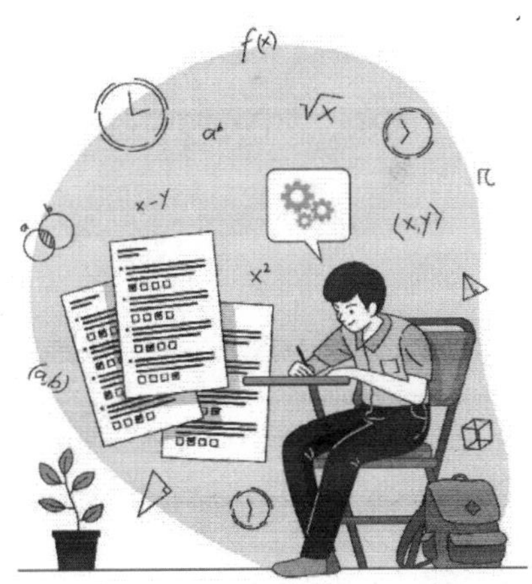

It's almost always better to start the guessing process too early than too late. It only takes a few seconds to remember something and answer the question from knowledge. Carefully eliminating wrong answer choices takes longer. Plus, going through the process of eliminating answer choices can actually help jog your memory.

Summary: Start the guessing process as soon as you decide that you can't answer the question based on your knowledge.

How to Narrow Down the Choices

The next chapter in this book (**Test-Taking Strategies**) includes a wide range of strategies for how to approach questions and how to look for answer choices to eliminate. You will definitely want to read those carefully, practice them, and figure out which ones work best for you. Here though, we're going to address a mindset rather than a particular strategy.

Your odds of guessing an answer correctly depend on how many options you are choosing from.

Number of options left	5	4	3	2	1
Odds of guessing correctly	20%	25%	33%	50%	100%

You can see from this chart just how valuable it is to be able to eliminate incorrect answers and make an educated guess, but there are two things that many test takers do that cause them to miss out on the benefits of guessing:

- Accidentally eliminating the correct answer
- Selecting an answer based on an impression

We'll look at the first one here, and the second one in the next section.

To avoid accidentally eliminating the correct answer, we recommend a thought exercise called **the $5 challenge**. In this challenge, you only eliminate an answer choice from contention if you are willing to bet $5 on it being wrong. Why $5? Five dollars is a small but not insignificant amount of money. It's an amount you could afford to lose but wouldn't want to throw away. And while losing $5 once might not hurt too much, doing it twenty times will set you back $100. In the same way, each small decision you make—eliminating a choice here, guessing on a question there—won't by itself impact your score very much, but when you put them all together, they can make a big difference. By holding each answer choice elimination decision to a higher standard, you can reduce the risk of accidentally eliminating the correct answer.

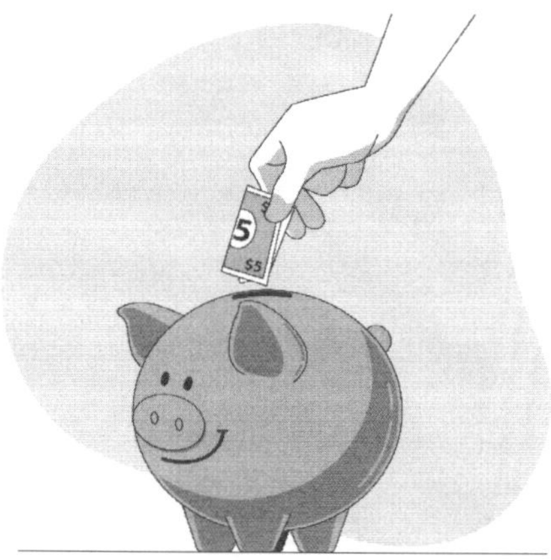

The $5 challenge can also be applied in a positive sense: If you are willing to bet $5 that an answer choice *is* correct, go ahead and mark it as correct.

Summary: Only eliminate an answer choice if you are willing to bet $5 that it is wrong.

Which Answer to Choose

You're taking the test. You've run into a hard question and decided you'll have to guess. You've eliminated all the answer choices you're willing to bet $5 on. Now you have to pick an answer. Why do we even need to talk about this? Why can't you just pick whichever one you feel like when the time comes?

The answer to these questions is that if you don't come into the test with a plan, you'll rely on your impression to select an answer choice, and if you do that, you risk falling into a trap. The test writers know that everyone who takes their test will be guessing on some of the questions, so they intentionally write wrong answer choices to seem plausible. You still have to pick an answer though, and if the wrong answer choices are designed to look right, how can you ever be sure that you're not falling for their trap? The best solution we've found to this dilemma is to take the decision out of your hands entirely. Here is the process we recommend:

Once you've eliminated any choices that you are confident (willing to bet $5) are wrong, select the first remaining choice as your answer.

Whether you choose to select the first remaining choice, the second, or the last, the important thing is that you use some preselected standard. Using this approach guarantees that you will not be enticed into selecting an answer choice that looks right, because you are not basing your decision on how the answer choices look.

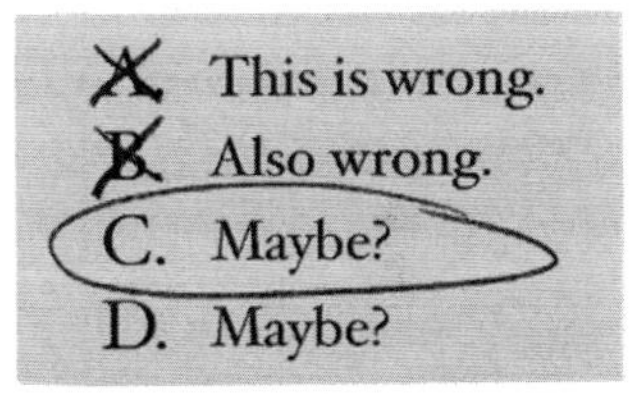

This is not meant to make you question your knowledge. Instead, it is to help you recognize the difference between your knowledge and your impressions. There's a huge difference between thinking an answer is right because of what you know, and thinking an answer is right because it looks or sounds like it should be right.

Summary: To ensure that your selection is appropriately random, make a predetermined selection from among all answer choices you have not eliminated.

Test-Taking Strategies

This section contains a list of test-taking strategies that you may find helpful as you work through the test. By taking what you know and applying logical thought, you can maximize your chances of answering any question correctly!

It is very important to realize that every question is different and every person is different: no single strategy will work on every question, and no single strategy will work for every person. That's why we've included all of them here, so you can try them out and determine which ones work best for different types of questions and which ones work best for you.

Question Strategies

☑ Read Carefully

Read the question and the answer choices carefully. Don't miss the question because you misread the terms. You have plenty of time to read each question thoroughly and make sure you understand what is being asked. Yet a happy medium must be attained, so don't waste too much time. You must read carefully and efficiently.

☑ Contextual Clues

Look for contextual clues. If the question includes a word you are not familiar with, look at the immediate context for some indication of what the word might mean. Contextual clues can often give you all the information you need to decipher the meaning of an unfamiliar word. Even if you can't determine the meaning, you may be able to narrow down the possibilities enough to make a solid guess at the answer to the question.

☑ Prefixes

If you're having trouble with a word in the question or answer choices, try dissecting it. Take advantage of every clue that the word might include. Prefixes can be a huge help. Usually, they allow you to determine a basic meaning. *Pre-* means before, *post-* means after, *pro-* is positive, *de-* is negative. From prefixes, you can get an idea of the general meaning of the word and try to put it into context.

☑ Hedge Words

Watch out for critical hedge words, such as *likely, may, can, often, almost, mostly, usually, generally, rarely,* and *sometimes.* Question writers insert these hedge phrases to cover every possibility. Often an answer choice will be wrong simply because it leaves no room for exception. Be on guard for answer choices that have definitive words such as *exactly* and *always.*

☑ Switchback Words

Stay alert for *switchbacks.* These are the words and phrases frequently used to alert you to shifts in thought. The most common switchback words are *but, although,* and *however.* Others include *nevertheless, on the other hand, even though, while, in spite of, despite,* and *regardless of.* Switchback words are important to catch because they can change the direction of the question or an answer choice.

⊘ Face Value

When in doubt, use common sense. Accept the situation in the problem at face value. Don't read too much into it. These problems will not require you to make wild assumptions. If you have to go beyond creativity and warp time or space in order to have an answer choice fit the question, then you should move on and consider the other answer choices. These are normal problems rooted in reality. The applicable relationship or explanation may not be readily apparent, but it is there for you to figure out. Use your common sense to interpret anything that isn't clear.

Answer Choice Strategies

⊘ Answer Selection

The most thorough way to pick an answer choice is to identify and eliminate wrong answers until only one is left, then confirm it is the correct answer. Sometimes an answer choice may immediately seem right, but be careful. The test writers will usually put more than one reasonable answer choice on each question, so take a second to read all of them and make sure that the other choices are not equally obvious. As long as you have time left, it is better to read every answer choice than to pick the first one that looks right without checking the others.

⊘ Answer Choice Families

An answer choice family consists of two (in rare cases, three) answer choices that are very similar in construction and cannot all be true at the same time. If you see two answer choices that are direct opposites or parallels, one of them is usually the correct answer. For instance, if one answer choice says that quantity x increases and another either says that quantity x decreases (opposite) or says that quantity y increases (parallel), then those answer choices would fall into the same family. An answer choice that doesn't match the construction of the answer choice family is more likely to be incorrect. Most questions will not have answer choice families, but when they do appear, you should be prepared to recognize them.

⊘ Eliminate Answers

Eliminate answer choices as soon as you realize they are wrong, but make sure you consider all possibilities. If you are eliminating answer choices and realize that the last one you are left with is also wrong, don't panic. Start over and consider each choice again. There may be something you missed the first time that you will realize on the second pass.

⊘ Avoid Fact Traps

Don't be distracted by an answer choice that is factually true but doesn't answer the question. You are looking for the choice that answers the question. Stay focused on what the question is asking for so you don't accidentally pick an answer that is true but incorrect. Always go back to the question and make sure the answer choice you've selected actually answers the question and is not merely a true statement.

⊘ Extreme Statements

In general, you should avoid answers that put forth extreme actions as standard practice or proclaim controversial ideas as established fact. An answer choice that states the "process should be used in certain situations, if…" is much more likely to be correct than one that states the "process should be discontinued completely." The first is a calm rational statement and doesn't even make a definitive, uncompromising stance, using a hedge word *if* to provide wiggle room, whereas the second choice is far more extreme.

✓ Benchmark

As you read through the answer choices and you come across one that seems to answer the question well, mentally select that answer choice. This is not your final answer, but it's the one that will help you evaluate the other answer choices. The one that you selected is your benchmark or standard for judging each of the other answer choices. Every other answer choice must be compared to your benchmark. That choice is correct until proven otherwise by another answer choice beating it. If you find a better answer, then that one becomes your new benchmark. Once you've decided that no other choice answers the question as well as your benchmark, you have your final answer.

✓ Predict the Answer

Before you even start looking at the answer choices, it is often best to try to predict the answer. When you come up with the answer on your own, it is easier to avoid distractions and traps because you will know exactly what to look for. The right answer choice is unlikely to be word-for-word what you came up with, but it should be a close match. Even if you are confident that you have the right answer, you should still take the time to read each option before moving on.

General Strategies

✓ Tough Questions

If you are stumped on a problem or it appears too hard or too difficult, don't waste time. Move on! Remember though, if you can quickly check for obviously incorrect answer choices, your chances of guessing correctly are greatly improved. Before you completely give up, at least try to knock out a couple of possible answers. Eliminate what you can and then guess at the remaining answer choices before moving on.

✓ Check Your Work

Since you will probably not know every term listed and the answer to every question, it is important that you get credit for the ones that you do know. Don't miss any questions through careless mistakes. If at all possible, try to take a second to look back over your answer selection and make sure you've selected the correct answer choice and haven't made a costly careless mistake (such as marking an answer choice that you didn't mean to mark). This quick double check should more than pay for itself in caught mistakes for the time it costs.

✓ Pace Yourself

It's easy to be overwhelmed when you're looking at a page full of questions; your mind is confused and full of random thoughts, and the clock is ticking down faster than you would like. Calm down and maintain the pace that you have set for yourself. Especially as you get down to the last few minutes of the test, don't let the small numbers on the clock make you panic. As long as you are on track by monitoring your pace, you are guaranteed to have time for each question.

✓ Don't Rush

It is very easy to make errors when you are in a hurry. Maintaining a fast pace in answering questions is pointless if it makes you miss questions that you would have gotten right otherwise. Test writers like to include distracting information and wrong answers that seem right. Taking a little extra time to avoid careless mistakes can make all the difference in your test score. Find a pace that allows you to be confident in the answers that you select.

⊘ Keep Moving

Panicking will not help you pass the test, so do your best to stay calm and keep moving. Taking deep breaths and going through the answer elimination steps you practiced can help to break through a stress barrier and keep your pace.

Final Notes

The combination of a solid foundation of content knowledge and the confidence that comes from practicing your plan for applying that knowledge is the key to maximizing your performance on test day. As your foundation of content knowledge is built up and strengthened, you'll find that the strategies included in this chapter become more and more effective in helping you quickly sift through the distractions and traps of the test to isolate the correct answer.

Now that you're preparing to move forward into the test content chapters of this book, be sure to keep your goal in mind. As you read, think about how you will be able to apply this information on the test. If you've already seen sample questions for the test and you have an idea of the question format and style, try to come up with questions of your own that you can answer based on what you're reading. This will give you valuable practice applying your knowledge in the same ways you can expect to on test day.

Good luck and good studying!

Nutrition Assessment and Diagnosis

Nutrition Screening

Nutrition screening is a process used to identify patients who are at risk for the development of nutrition-related issues. Identifying these patients as having risk factors for nutritional issues allows the patient to receive a more in-depth nutrition assessment by a registered dietitian. The Patient Generated Subjective Global Assessment (PG-SGA) is a valid and reliable tool used in the nutrition screening process. The patient completes the first four sections, answering questions regarding weight status, food intake, types of symptoms being experienced, and information about daily activities. The health care professional then completes the remainder of the form, which explores current diagnosis and past history. The questionnaire is scored and the patient is determined to be either well nourished, with moderate or suspected malnutrition, or severely malnourished, which then determines the type of additional nutrition intervention required. This ranges from no intervention, management of symptoms, dietitian intervention, or more intensive intervention to address more critical issues.

Dietary History

Dietary history is an important component in the nutritional assessment of a patient with cancer. Essential information that should be obtained includes weight history and recent weight loss or gain, changes in appetite, presence of early satiety, food allergies and intolerances, and typical diet and food intake, including any deviation from normal. The diet history should also include information on the patient's functional status, such as the ability to work, prepare and shop for food, etc. Information on the use of any nutritional supplements or products, medication use, vitamin and mineral use, and the use of herbs or botanicals should also be obtained. Social factors that should be explored include support system, financial constraints, and religious or cultural issues that may have an impact on nutritional status. The use of alcohol and tobacco should also be determined. Aspects of the current disease process should also be explored, including treatment, symptoms, and side effects. A history of prior nutrition education should also be determined.

Physical Examination

A physical examination is extremely useful for assessing the nutritional status of a patient with cancer. The overall general appearance of the patient should be considered initially. This would include a visual assessment of size and frame. A visual assessment of functional status is also useful in terms of the patient's ability to ambulate and complete activities of daily life. A closer examination of certain areas of the body should be completed to aid in assessment. The face, especially the mouth area, can be examined for temporal wasting and evidence of vitamin deficiencies. Muscle mass and fat stores can be further evaluated if evidence of fat or muscle wasting is seen or if the rib cage, shoulder blade, or spine is protruding. The skin should be checked, as many vitamin and mineral deficiencies can be detected. Fluid status can also be assessed for dehydration, as evidenced by dry mucous membranes, or edema, as evidenced by puffiness in certain areas such as the ankle.

Anthropometrics

Anthropometric measurements are an important component of a comprehensive nutrition assessment. An accurate weight and height should be documented at start of treatment and should then be evaluated on the same scale at each office visit. Weight alterations need to be further evaluated, as maintaining a normal weight will help to promote a better outcome from cancer treatment. The National Cancer Institute Common Toxicity Criteria assess weight loss according to the following grades: Grade 0 or less than 5% weight loss, Grade 1, or weight loss of between 5 and 9.9%, Grade 2, or between 10 and 19.9% weight loss, and Grade 3, or greater than 20% weight loss. These criteria require updating, as weight loss should not exceed 20% in order to be considered serious. Other types of measurements that may be useful include triceps skinfold assessment to evaluate fat stores and mid-arm muscle circumference to evaluate muscle mass and protein stores. Standards are widely available for comparison; however, because these standards are derived from healthy individuals without a cancer diagnosis, their use is often limited in patients with cancer.

DIETARY SUPPLEMENTS

The use of dietary supplements such as vitamins, herbs, or botanicals is increasing in popularity every year. If a patient is considering using any of these products, it is imperative for him or her to fully understand the potential implications. This decision should be weighed carefully and made with the guidance of the physician treating the patient. The FDA has established regulations to help with the safety of these products, but full implementation will not occur until 2010. Fully understanding the risks and side effects of these products regarding dosage and potential interactions with other medications is necessary. The patient should also understand that a product labeled as natural does not necessarily make it safer to use. Products should be from a reputable manufacturer that uses good quality control practices. The generic or cheaper version of a product is not usually the best choice.

FDA REGULATIONS

The Dietary Supplement Health and Education Act (DSHEA) in 1994 began to categorize dietary supplements as a food; as such, these supplements are subject to a different set of rules than drugs. Dietary supplements were generally considered safe unless proven to be harmful. Thus, manufacturers were not required to test any new ingredient in a clinical trial to determine any harmful side effects, which were usually discovered after a patient experienced an adverse reaction to the dietary supplement or new ingredient. Starting in 2007 and ending in 2010, more stringent requirements are being implemented requiring companies that manufacture dietary supplements to follow Good Manufacturing Practices, ensuring that quality control is in place, the product does not contain any impurities, and the label is truthful. These regulations do not control the safety of the ingredients in the product nor do they control the effects on the physical health of the consumer. Even with the new regulations, problems can still exist with dietary supplements.

NON-TRADITIONAL PHARMACOLOGICAL AND BIOLOGICAL CANCER TREATMENTS

There are many examples of non-traditional pharmacological and biological treatment methods for cancer. The majority of these treatments is considered experimental and is not usually recognized by traditional medicine. Many may cause potentially dangerous reactions. The American Cancer Society website has a full listing of potential treatments. Examples include:

- Apiotherapy-- products obtained from honey bees thought to have anti-tumor properties
- Di Bella Therapy-- a mixture of the drugs somatostatin and bromocriptine along with vitamins, minerals, melatonin, and possibly certain chemotherapy drugs. The mixture is supposed to shrink tumors and promote self healing; however, the claims have not been substantiated.
- Laetrile-- a product made from the pits of apricots, peaches, and almonds used as a form of chemotherapy. The use of this can possibly cause cyanide toxicity.
- Shark cartilage-- a product obtained from the heads and fins of sharks thought to slow cancer progression by cutting off the blood supply to the tumor. Evidence does not support its effectiveness.

ALTERNATIVE DIET AND NUTRITION THERAPIES

The following are alternative diet and nutrition therapies:

- Fasting-- this therapy involves abstaining from any type of food for up to 5 days as part of a detoxification process. Water and juice may be consumed. This type of alternative metabolic therapy is thought to remove harmful substances from the body in order to allow the body to focus on healing itself of the cancer. Some also believe that fasting will starve the tumor, causing the cancer cells to die. This is not supported by mainstream medicine, as it may interfere with weight maintenance and the consumption of a healthy diet.
- Garlic-- studies are being conducted to evaluate the benefit of large doses of garlic on cancer. Garlic may contain immune properties that may slow cancer growth. Initial studies suggest that the use of garlic may lower the risk of stomach, prostate, and colon cancer. Possible side effects include stomachache or gas. It may also affect bleeding due to anti-clotting factors.
- Gerson Therapy-- a form of metabolic therapy involving the use of coffee enemas coupled with a special vegetarian diet and certain supplements such as vitamin B12, potassium, and pancreatic enzymes. The patient is expected to consume up to 20 pounds of fresh fruits and vegetables every day. It is thought to help detoxify the body and improve immune function and metabolism. The only licensed clinic available is in Mexico. It is a potentially dangerous therapy for a patient with cancer to follow, as the coffee enemas may lead to electrolyte depletion and the constant use of enemas may cause problems with the colon. Other complications are possible as well.
- Juicing-- involves processing fruits and vegetables in order to obtain the juices thought to improve the immune system and cleanse the body of toxins. The removal of the pulp also removes the benefit of the fiber. Overall, the process of juicing is not thought to be harmful if consumed as part of a regular diet for most people.
- Acidophilus-- a probiotic and considered helpful in maintaining normal gut flora. It is thought to help prevent certain types of cancer such as colon cancer by offsetting other carcinogens in the diet. Although the purported cancer-fighting benefits of this product have not been demonstrated in large clinical trials, it is rarely harmful if used as an adjunct to traditional therapy.
- Lycopene-- an antioxidant found in tomatoes. People whose diets include lycopene may have a lower risk of cancer, although further research is warranted.
- Macrobiotic diet-- A macrobiotic diet is a type of vegetarian diet derived from ancient Asian traditions. The diet portion itself is not dangerous, as it promotes a lower fat and higher fiber intake that can have positive impact on overall health. Proper diet planning is important to make sure it is nutritionally sound. In the past, more extreme forms of the diet were practiced that were dangerous. The diet consists of 50% to 60% organic whole grains, 20% to 25% organic fruits and vegetables, and 5% to 10% soup made from seaweed, beans, certain grains, and miso. Red meat, poultry, eggs, coffee, dairy, sugar, and processed foods are avoided. The food is prepared in certain types of cookware such as wood, glass, or stainless steel. Microwaves are avoided and many people also avoid cooking with electricity. Research is being conducted to explore the benefits of this diet for treating or curing cancer.
- Sea vegetables-- types of algae and seaweed thought to contain special nutrients that revive the body and improve thyroid function and weight. It is also thought to lower the risk of breast cancer, although it is difficult to pinpoint if seaweed is actually the reason for this. Many types of seaweed are edible; however, because some types are toxic and may even cause death, extreme caution needs to be taken.

- Omega 3 fatty acids-- fatty acids that are not made by the body but are essential to many functions of the body. The belief is that omega 3 fatty acids help to stop the spread of cancers that are influenced by hormones such as breast cancer. It is also thought to stop the growth of prostate, colon, and pancreatic tumors. The evidence for these claims is not as strong as it is for its other benefits such as reducing cardiac risk factors. Risks involve high doses interfering with normal blood clotting, which may also increase total cholesterol.
- Quercetin-- a phytochemical found in apples, red wine, onions, and other foods as well as in supplement form. Quercetin is thought to promote antihistamine effects as well as antioxidant and anti-inflammatory effects. The research is not conclusive at this time but it is recommended that these food items be included as part of a normal diet.
- Soybeans-- thought to possess protective properties against certain types of cancer including breast, prostate, lung, and colon. The properties are thought to be due to isoflavones or phytoestrogens. The results of research on the actual benefits are mixed, and may be related to age or other factors. The use of soybeans is safe for most people.
- Vegetarianism-- a type of dietary practice that involves ingesting foods derived from plant sources. Animal products are usually avoided, although some people may include dairy, fish, or eggs. The belief for this practice is that a healthy, plant-based diet promotes general good health and is protective against cancer. Caution must be taken to include sources of all vitamins and minerals to prevent deficiencies, especially of vitamins B12 and D, calcium, iron, and zinc. Adequate calorie intake is also essential to maintain weight for those with cancer.
- Wheatgrass-- a type of grass found in milder climates that are usually ingested in the form of a juice. The belief is that wheatgrass improves immune function and causes tumors to shrink and improves mortality for patients with cancer. No research on humans has been completed to document its effectiveness. It is not considered to be dangerous, but some side effects may be experienced such as nausea, headaches, or an anaphylactic reaction in a few people.
- Willard water-- also known as catalyst-altered water. It is a type of water that contains calcium and magnesium as well as castor oil. It is considered to have an electric charge and is supposed to relieve mouth pain form sores or radiation therapy. It is also reported to help with digestion and absorption. No studies have been completed and its safety has not been determined.

Mind, Body, and Spirit in Cancer Treatment

Research has shown that a good, positive attitude coupled with a determined spirit can have a positive effect on the body's response to cancer treatment. The effects can range from improvement in immune function to improvements in emotional status and physical health. There are many types of treatments offered in the realm of mind, body, and spirit. This type of treatment is also known as psychoneuroimmunology (PNI). Examples of this type of therapy include aromatherapy, bioenergetics, breathwork, cymatic therapy, faith healing, humor therapy, and hypnosis. Other examples include dance therapy, imagery, meditation, Native American healing, psychotherapy, qigong, and tai chi.

Alternative and Complementary Medicines

Alternative medicine and complementary medicine are very different concepts. Alternative medicine is used in place of standardized medical care. This can often have disastrous results in terms of adversely affecting prognosis and life expectancy. Complementary medicine is used in conjunction with standardized medical treatment. This is referred to as integrative therapy. The majority of complementary treatments are safe, but some may be capable of causing harm; thus, patients should be careful when making the decision to utilize a complementary treatment. Some patients may opt to try either of these treatments but must be aware of the risks involved. Some patients want to try something in order to treat the side effects of cancer treatment but do not want to ingest additional medications. Other people may prefer nontraditional medicine and feel they are making the correct choice for themselves. Others may try a treatment that may have fewer side effects, while still others may want to try to improve their overall health status.

Although traditional cancer treatments are the recommended course of treatment for the majority of patients, complementary medicine may be a good alternative to help relieve the side effects of treatment, for pain control, or for an overall improved sense of well-being. Any decision should be discussed with the attending physician to ensure safety. Available complementary therapies include massage therapy, meditation, art therapy, spirituality, yoga, aromatherapy, acupuncture, and music therapy. The patient should be suspicious of any therapy that advocates complete cure, is based on unproven methods, is only offered by one clinic, requires international travel, and advises against using traditional medical treatments. Other considerations include how the therapy is advertised and the cost of treatment.

Refeeding syndrome

Refeeding syndrome can occur when concentrated nutrition is provided in a rapid manner to a patient who has malnutrition; this sets off a series of metabolic consequences that can seriously endanger a patient's life. Hyperglycemia develops, which may lead to hypophosphatemia, hypokalemia, and hypomagnesemia as the electrolytes shift from extracellular to intracellular spaces. This syndrome will typically occur within the first 5 days of initiating nutrition support. Severe alterations in cardiac function may occur for several reasons: First, the heart is often atrophied due to the malnourished state; secondly, increased stress is placed on the weakened heart as the volume status rapidly expands and the heart muscle has difficulty handling the excess fluid. This additional fluid may cause respiratory failure. Neurologic alterations are also possible due in part to the electrolyte abnormalities. Other complications can include gastrointestinal alterations such as diarrhea, constipation, or abdominal pain. Hematologic complications are also possible such as anemia, thrombocytopenia, or decreased platelet function.

Cancer staging

Staging is defined as determining the extent of the cancer and exactly where it is located. This information enables the physician to develop a plan of care for treating the patient and provides information about expected prognosis. Staging is based on three factors and uses a system called TNM staging: T refers to the size of the primary tumor and if the tumor has invaded other areas close to the primary site, N refers to whether the tumor has spread into the lymph nodes, and M refers to whether the cancer has spread to other areas of the body. Tests such as CT scans, x-rays, MRI, and biopsies are often used to gather this information. Staging does not change from diagnosis but as the cancer progresses; additional information is obtained according to the current status of the cancer.

Tumor markers

Tumor markers are usually a type of protein that is found in the body indicating that cancer is present. Tumor markers are typically found in the blood or urine. Tumor markers are used for screening and for early detection of certain types of cancer. The most commonly used tumor marker is prostate-specific antigen (PSA) for the detection of prostate cancer. Tumor markers are not diagnostic in nature but can be indicative of whether a cancer is present. Some tumor markers can be used to gauge whether a certain cancer is aggressive. Other markers can help to monitor the effectiveness of cancer treatment. If the tumor marker decreases, this most often indicates that the cancer is responding to treatment. Tumor markers can also be used to monitor cancer recurrence, although most physicians do not rely solely on this method for determining if a cancer has returned.

Diagnostic procedures

Diagnostic procedures are listed and described below:

- Fine needle aspiration-- uses a very thin needle that is inserted into the tumor; fluid or tissue is withdrawn into a syringe. This is often conducted using an ultrasound or CT scan. An incision is not needed for this procedure.
- Core needle biopsy-- involves the use of a larger needle to remove a tissue sample; a larger sample can be obtained. This type of procedure may also be used with ultrasound or CT scan for guidance.
- Excisional biopsy-- involves the removal of the whole tumor through a small incision in the skin; an incisional biopsy involves the partial removal of a tumor. This procedure can be done using local or general anesthesia depending upon the location of the tumor.
- Ultrasound-- involves the use of high-frequency sound waves to observe organs and tissues within the body
- Laparoscopy-- a fine tube inserted through an incision in the abdomen to visualize the pelvic region and abdomen.
- Thoracoscopy-- a fine tube used to visualize the inside of the chest and pleural cavity
- Mediastinoscopy- a fine tube inserted through the neck used to visualize the inside of the mediastinum (the space between the pleural sacs)
- Laparotomy, thoracotomy, and mediastinotomy-- types of open surgery in which a small incision is made under general anesthesia in order for the surgeon to better visualize the area being examined. Laparotomy is conducted in the abdominal area, thoracotomy in the area between the lungs and chest wall, and mediastinotomy in the area between the lungs
- Thoracentesis-- a needle is placed in the area around the ribs to obtain a fluid sample and drain any fluid that is present
- Endoscopy-- a procedure that utilizes a long, thin tube with fiber optics for visualizing the inside of the body. Some endoscopes include cameras, and biopsies can often be obtained if necessary. The main purpose of endoscopy is for diagnosis. This procedure can be done using either general or local anesthesia. Types of endoscopies include:
    - Sigmoidoscopy-- visualizes the rectum and lower part of the large intestine to detect signs of cancer or polyps. Polyps can eventually become cancerous.
    - Colonoscopy-- visualizes the large intestine.
    - Esophagogastroduodenoscopy-- also known as EGD. This visualizes the esophagus, stomach, and duodenum.
- Barium enema-- a type of procedure used to diagnose colorectal cancer. Barium is ingested by the patient in order for the colon to be visualized on x-ray.
- Upper GI series-- a procedure in which the patient ingests barium to visualize the lining of the esophagus, stomach, and duodenum using x-rays.

Cytology

Cytology is a way to diagnose a disease by looking at single cells or a cluster of cells. Cytology is less invasive than a biopsy. A cytology sample is usually obtained using fine-needle aspiration biopsy. The types of fluids that are tested may include blood, urine, sputum, pleural fluid, pericardial fluid, spinal fluid, or fluid from ascites. Cells can also be obtained by gently scraping off tissue, such as in a Pap test. The pathologist observes the gross appearance of the sample and also examines the specimen under a microscope. Sometimes the samples are treated with a type of stain or are concentrated before they can be examined. Some cancers such as adenocarcinoma or osteosarcomas can be classified using cytology. Cancers can also be graded as high- or low-grade, which can help to determine the prognosis of the patient.

Pathology

Pathology is defined as any deviation in anatomy or physiology from normal standards that would indicate disease or be characteristic of a certain disease. A pathology report is the essential piece for planning treatment. Generally the pathology report contains the patient's name and identifying number, name of the doctor, and type of specimen used for cytology. The report will also contain past medical history of the patient and any noteworthy information included by the doctor who obtained the sample. The report will also contain the gross description, or the description that can be given based on what is seen without a microscope; it also contains information about what is seen through the microscope, such as the presence or arrangement of cancer cells. The diagnosis is made through the pathology report and is based on the results of all the testing performed on the sample. There is also a section for comments from the pathologist and a general summary of all the findings that should be significant for planning treatment.

Oral or Oropharyngeal Cancer

Symptoms and Diagnosis

Common symptoms of oral cancer are a nonhealing sore inside the mouth, a lump in the area of the cheeks or neck, unexplained mouth pain, or red or white patches inside the mouth, on the gums or tongue, or on the tonsils. Other symptoms include difficulty chewing or swallowing, pain in the jaw area, numbness inside the mouth, loose teeth, ongoing breath issues, and weight loss. To diagnose cancer in the oral or oropharyngeal regions, the physician does a complete physical examination. A referral to an ears, nose, and throat (ENT) specialist or a surgeon specializing in maxillofacial surgery may be recommended. Possible tests include nasopharyngoscopy, pharyngoscopy, or laryngoscopy. A biopsy is done in the doctor's office or in the operating room under anesthesia if the tumor is difficult to access, or using fine needle aspiration. Possible imaging tests include chest x-rays, CT scans, or magnetic resonance imaging (MRI). A barium swallow is often done to obtain further diagnostic information.

Surgeries

The following are types of oral or oropharyngeal surgeries:

- Primary tumor resection-- the removal of the whole tumor along with surrounding tissue to lessen the chance of cancer cells being missed. This procedure can be done through the mouth for smaller tumors or through the neck for larger tumors. Sometimes the jaw bone must be cut to get to the tumor.
- Maxillectomy-- the removal of the maxilla bone for cancers related to the hard palate, including the roof of the mouth.
- Neck dissection-- there are three types of neck dissections. Partial neck dissection involves the removal of a limited number of lymph nodes. A modified radical neck dissection involves the removal of lymph nodes located on one side of the neck between the jaw and clavicle; muscle and nerve tissue are also removed. A radical neck dissection involves the removal of all of the lymph nodes plus additional muscles, nerve tissue, and veins; it is a much more invasive procedure.

Head and Neck Cancer

Patients with cancer of the head and neck typically experience dysphagia, which usually worsens as the cancer progresses. This type of cancer results in a longer oral and pharyngeal phase of swallowing and overall less efficient swallowing. The size of the tumor is directly related to swallow impairment. Patients with head and neck cancer may be dealing with the after-effects of surgical resection. Patients who have had resections such as mandibulectomy, glossectomy, or resection of the hard palate or lips will experience defects in the oral preparation or propulsion phase of swallowing. The pharyngeal phase of swallow can be affected by surgeries such as laryngectomy, pharyngolaryngectomy, tracheotomy, or any surgery of the soft palate region. It can also be affected by any disorder of the pharynx, weakened pharyngeal muscles, or oropharyngeal surgery. Altered body image coupled with changes in ability to eat can also lead to fear of eating with others.

Patients with head and neck cancer often develop side effects following treatment. Radiation therapy is a common treatment modality for these patients and dysphagia and odynophagia can develop during the course of treatment. Additionally, xerostomia can develop because of targeted radiation to the area that holds the salivary glands. Xerostomia can interfere with normal bolus formation. Ongoing fungal infections are also a possibility due to chronic inflammation and reduced immunity from the lack of saliva. Various types of resections such as laryngectomies can be associated with a higher risk of aspiration due to altered swallow function following the procedure. Patients who have had glossectomies also have difficulty forming boluses of food and fluids, increasing the risk for aspiration as well. Resection of the mandibular area can cause problems with chewing. Patients who have had a tracheostomy may experience difficulty swallowing due to the location of the procedure.

Cancer of the Esophagus

After diagnosing cancer of the esophagus, the cancer is staged. Treatment may involve surgery. The two most common types of surgeries are esophagectomy, which is the removal of part of the esophagus and lymph nodes. The esophagus is attached directly to the stomach or may be attached via a piece of the intestines. An esophagogastrectomy is another type of surgery involving the removal of the lower esophagus, lymph nodes, and the upper portion of the stomach. The esophagus is reattached to the remaining part of the stomach. Many times, a feeding tube is placed during the procedure to aid in postoperative nutrition. Chemotherapy and radiation therapy are often done in conjunction with surgery to help relieve symptoms but are not necessarily curative on their own.

Esophageal Cancer

The two most common types of esophageal cancer are squamous cell or adenocarcinoma. Squamous cell cancer can present at any point along the entire length of the esophagus, whereas adenocarcinoma typically presents in the lower portion of the esophagus. The two most common risk factors for developing esophageal cancer are the use of tobacco and alcohol. The main treatment for patients with esophageal cancer is an esophagectomy. Many times chemotherapy and/or radiation therapy are also required. Complications from this type of surgery may include strictures, dysmotility, leaks at the anastomotic site, bleeding, infection, and injury to laryngeal nerves.

Pancreatic Cancer

Weight loss is the most common presenting symptom of a patient with pancreatic cancer. Often these patients have lost as much as 15% of pre-illness weight when they are diagnosed. Malabsorption may also be seen as a result of pancreatic enzyme deficiency. The tumor may obstruct the common bile duct, leading to bile insufficiency with nutritional deficiencies; hyperglycemia is often seen as well. Pancreatic cancer is most often located in the pancreatic duct or the head of the pancreas. Surgery is the best curative option; however, many patients are not able to undergo surgery because the cancer has already spread. Some patients will receive surgery as a palliative measure or will receive chemoradiation in hopes of shrinking the tumor before surgery. The most common surgery used for patients with pancreatic cancer is a pancreaticoduodenectomy, also known as a Whipple procedure. In this procedure, the head of the pancreas, the duodenum, the distal stomach, and part of the bile duct are removed. There is also a variation known as a pylorus-preserving pancreatoduodenectomy (PPPD) where the distal portion of the stomach is not removed. Potential complications of the Whipple procedure include dumping syndrome, delayed gastric emptying, leak at the anastomotic site, diarrhea, early satiety, and ulceration due to bile acid reflux. Most patients require gastric decompression following surgery. If the PPPD is performed instead, the risk of developing dumping syndrome and ulceration at the stoma is reduced.

Colorectal Cancer

Surgery is generally the treatment used to treat colorectal cancers. The types of surgeries that may be performed will vary based on the location of the tumor but may include a colectomy and possibly lymph node resection for polyps that have invaded the vascular system or that contain poorly differentiated cells. For cancers of the colon and the top third of the rectum, a tumor resection with a primary anastomosis is typically performed. Rectal cancer surgery often involves a colostomy or an ileostomy. A permanent colostomy will be required if the anal sphincter muscles and rectum are resected or removed.

Types of Surgeries Performed and Associated Terms Are as Follows:

- Polypectomy--the removal of polyps during a colonoscopy
- Right colectomy-- the removal of the right side of the colon. Sometimes the ileum is also removed (called an ileocolectomy) because the ileum is located at the right side of the colon.
- Proctosigmoidectomy-- the removal of the sigmoid colon and the diseased portion of the rectum.
- Total colectomy-- removal of the entire colon; the rectum and anus are left intact.
- Total proctocolectomy- the removal of both the colon and the rectum. If the anus is also removed, an ileal pouch will be created in order to remove waste. If the anus is removed, a permanent ileostomy is created.
- Stoma-- an opening in the skin or bowel
- Temporary stoma-- an opening created to divert stool away from the damaged bowel or away from the portion that was recently resected to allow for healing to occur. A temporary colostomy can usually be reversed in 8 to12 weeks depending upon the healing process, presence of other chronic diseases, and overall current state of health.
- Permanent stoma-- an opening created to make permanent diversion for stool to pass
- Colostomy-- an opening of the colon through the skin used for the removal of stool from the body
- Ileostomy-- an opening of the ileum, which is part of the small intestine, through the skin.

Cancer Surgeries

The following types of general cancer surgeries:

- Preventive surgery-- involves the removal of a certain type of tissue that may become cancerous at a later time. An example of this is removal of polyps in the colon before they become cancerous.
- Diagnostic surgery-- involves the use of surgery to obtain a biopsy in order to determine if the tissue involved is cancerous

- Staging surgery-- involves the use of surgery to determine the extent of the cancer and whether it has spread to other organs
- Curative surgery-- the removal of an entire tumor that involves only one area. This can be used in conjunction with chemotherapy and/or radiation therapy.
- Debulking surgery-- involves the removal of a portion of a tumor, usually for advanced stages of cancer. This may be done because removal of the entire tumor may be dangerous to other organs and tissue that are near the site of the tumor. This is most often used in conjunction with chemotherapy and/or radiation therapy.
- Palliative surgery-- involves advanced stages of cancer and is not done as a curative measure. It is used for relief of discomfort or for pain relief.
- Supportive surgery-- used for adjunct therapy such as the placement of a catheter for chemotherapy.
- Restorative surgery-- also called reconstructive therapy. This involves correction of the results of a prior surgery for purposes of aesthetics or organ function. An example of this would be mandibular reconstructive surgery using bone grafts, tissue flaps, or prosthetic devices.

SURGERY RELATED NUTRITION ISSUES

The following surgeries may cause nutrition-related issues or nutrient deficiencies:

- Esophagectomy-- can cause early satiety, regurgitation, or diarrhea/steatorrhea due to vagotomy.
- Gastrectomy-- a total resection can cause early satiety due to removal of reservoir, as well as malabsorption, dumping syndrome, vitamin B12 deficiency due to loss of intrinsic factors, and hypoglycemia.
- Jejunal or ileal resection-- has the potential to cause multiple nutrient deficiencies such as vitamin B12, calcium, magnesium, and fat malabsorption, along with malabsorption of fat-soluble vitamins. This type of resection may also cause kidney stones due to hyperoxaluria.
- Ileostomy or colostomy-- can cause problems with salt and water balance and malabsorption.
- Massive bowel resection-- this type of resection has the potential to cause major malnutrition due to malabsorption. It can also cause metabolic acidosis, dehydration, and can be life-threatening.

PEDIATRIC ACUTE LYMPHOCYTIC LEUKEMIA

There are generally three phases of chemotherapy required for a child diagnosed with acute lymphocytic leukemia (ALL): induction, consolidation, and maintenance. Induction chemotherapy is given with the goal of achieving remission, which may occur within the first month of treatment. The 3 drugs most often used together are L-asparaginase, vincristine, and a form of steroid such as dexamethasone. Consolidation chemotherapy is in the most intensive phase, lasting up to 8 months. The goal of this phase is to reduce the number of leukemia cells that are still in the body. The drugs used in this phase may vary but may include methotrexate or 6-mercaptopurine. Maintenance chemotherapy begins after the maintenance phase ends; the goal of this phase is to prevent recurrence of ALL. The drugs used may include methotrexate and 6-mercaptopurine as well as vincristine and another steroid. These drugs are given every 1 to 2 months. The length of time required for all three phases is between 2 and 3 years and the survival rate is 80%.

Pediatric Medulloblastoma

Screening tools for central nervous system tumors do not exist. Instead, symptoms such as nausea and vomiting may be present when the child goes from sitting to standing. Other symptoms may include a sudden change in vision, changes in speech, loss of memory, and difficulty with balance. Surgery is the primary treatment for brain tumors such as medulloblastoma if the tumor is easy to resect. Some tumors are able to be completely removed while others are not. For those tumors that are deeply embedded in the brain, debulking may be performed, which will reduce the size of the tumor. Typically, both radiation and chemotherapy are used in conjunction with surgery. Other medications that may be used include corticosteroids such as dexamethasone for reducing the amount of brain swelling, diuretics such as mannitol for reducing brain swelling and pressure, pain medications, and anti-seizure medications such as phenytoin.

Implications of Malnutrition in Surgical Oncology

Surgery is the primary treatment method for many types of cancers. Surgery itself can cause side effects such as increased fatigue, changes in appetite, increased calorie and protein requirements for healing, and changes in bowel function related to the use of anesthesia or pain medication. Individuals who have a dual diagnosis of cancer requiring surgery and malnutrition are at even higher risk for complications. The ability to tolerate a surgical procedure is impaired and morbidity and mortality rates are increased. Preoperative enteral nutrition support should be initiated for any patient who is severely malnourished. Other malnourished patients who should receive preoperative enteral nutrition include those who can have surgery delayed for at least a week and those in whom clinical improvement has been documented due to the use of nutrition support. The main goal of preoperative enteral nutrition is to prevent or slow further weight loss and prevent nutrient deficiencies from developing or worsening.

HSCT

The first step in the HSCT (hematopoietic stem cell transplant) process is to determine eligibility for a transplant. HLA tissue typing occurs, along with a complete medical, psychological, and social evaluation. Consultation with the transplant team is arranged. Many procedures may be done, such as CT scans or pulmonary tests; lab work is completed. Issues that must be considered are possible outcomes without transplant, complications related to the procedure, possible recurrence following transplant, and possible side effects of the procedure. Other issues to be explored include financial, housing options if the treatment center is located away from home, family support while the patient is away, and the selection of the donor. A central venous catheter may be placed for medication access or blood draws. The evaluation will determine if the transplant will be done in the hospital or as an outpatient. Inpatient programs provide rooms with specialized air filtration systems to help protect the patient from outside air and possible infection.

Conditioning and Transplant Phases

The actual transplant process starts in the conditioning phase, with chemotherapy and/or radiation therapy. This phase usually lasts for 7 to10 days. Side effects are most likely due to the effects of the treatment and may occur on the day of conditioning when treatment is administered. Possible side effects include nausea, vomiting, diarrhea, and loss of appetite; mucositis may start as well. The transplant phase begins with an infusion of either bone marrow or peripheral blood stem cells through the central catheter. The day this occurs is called Day zero. Side effects during this phase are not common, and if present, are usually mild.

Recovery Phase

The neutropenic phase is part of the recovery phase and may last 2 to 4 weeks. This phase consists mainly of waiting for the immune system to recover and encompasses intensive monitoring and support, along with the management of complications. This phase is often the most stressful for patients, as it involves a lot of waiting and hoping. The risk for infection is high, and steps must be taken to prevent infection from occurring. The next part is the engraftment and early recovery phase. This occurs anywhere from 10 to 28 days following transplant and is evidenced by new bone marrow or stem cell production indicative of an immune system that is trying to recover. Intensive monitoring continues, but the patient may be eligible for discharge during this phase.

Discharge

The last phase is discharge, which may occur when the neutrophil count is over 500/mm^3, the patient has been afebrile for at least 48 hours, and side effects such as nausea or vomiting are well controlled. The hematocrit level must be at least 25% and platelets must be greater than 15,000/mm^3. The patient must be able to take all medication by mouth and be able to tolerate an oral diet. Adequate supports must be in place at home. The actual discharge planning process should begin when the patient is admitted. Education is intense and completed by the various members of the transplant team. Instructions include diet and nutrition education, catheter care, and follow-up instructions. Rehabilitation can last up to a year. Sometimes frequent lab work is indicated and possibly blood or platelet transfusions. Complications can occur after HSCT such as graft vs. host disease, infections, thyroid issues, other types of cancer, fatigue, or personal issues.

GVHD

GVHD (acute graft versus host disease) is a condition that may occur in patients who have had allogeneic stem cell transplants. The donor cells believe that the recipient's body is foreign and begin to attack certain organs such as the skin, GI tract, or liver. This is a very common occurrence and the severity can range from mild to very severe. It will mainly occur between 3 and 4 weeks posttransplant, but can occur anywhere between 10 to 70 days following the procedure. Symptoms may include a burning rash and redness of the hands and feet. Other symptoms include nausea, vomiting, abdominal pain, jaundice, or poor appetite. Medications are generally provided to patients posttransplant to help prevent this from occurring, although milder cases of GVHD are still common. The medications provided include steroids, methotrexate, cyclosporine, and tacrolimus.

Chronic GVHD is an ongoing condition that may develop after 3 months and up to 400 days following stem cell transplant. The first sign is usually a rash on the hands or bottoms of the feet. The rash may worsen to the point of blistering and peeling. Symptoms of chronic GVHD include poor appetite and weight loss, diarrhea, stomach pain, enlarged liver, and increased liver enzyme tests. Other symptoms may include dry eyes, painful mouth with sores present, and pain when eating highly acidic foods. Less common symptoms can include thinning of the hair. The medications that are used to treat this condition include steroids such as prednisone and cyclosporine.

Nutritional complications following Whipple procedure

As many as 25% of patients who undergo a Whipple procedure will experience malabsorption because of a deficiency of exocrine pancreatic enzymes, leading to Dumping Syndrome, In this situation, pancreatic enzyme replacement therapy should be initiated. Pancreatic lipase is prescribed to be taken at each meal and snack to aid in the absorption of fat. Calcium and the fat-soluble Vitamins A, D, E and K may also be indicated. Diabetes is also another potential complication because of the removal of the head of the pancreas, but is more serious for those patients who already have diabetes or glucose intolerance. Weight loss is also common postsurgery.

Signs and Symptoms of Cancer

Patients who are experiencing unexplained signs and symptoms will typically seek medical attention. It is important for the health care practitioner to differentiate between signs and symptoms but both are usually evaluated at the same time. Signs are objective issues pointing towards a disease process and can be measured in a quantitative manner. Examples of signs may be fever or rapid breathing. Symptoms, on the other hand, are subjective and often complicated. Symptoms are suggestive of an internal issue; however, symptoms do not typically provide concrete answers. Examples of symptoms may be weight loss, fatigue, or weakness. General signs and symptoms of cancer are often nonspecific and can also be associated with other disease processes, but should always be thoroughly evaluated by a physician. These include unexplained weight loss, pain, fever, fatigue, and abnormal change in skin condition such as color. More specific signs and symptoms include nonhealing skin lesions, changes in elimination habits, the discovery of a lump, abnormal bleeding, dysphagia, or prolonged cough.

Symptom Management

It is very important for health care practitioners to identify and address signs and symptoms that a patient may be experiencing. Failure to do so can significantly impact the quality of life and functional status of the patient. Uncontrolled signs and symptoms can also interfere with cancer treatment; however, there is a way to help a patient to describe exactly what he or she is feeling related to the symptom. Seven attributes have been identified, including the location, quality, and severity of the symptom, how often it occurs, the type of setting in which it most frequently occurs, factors that improve or worsen the symptom, and any other associated symptoms. The level of symptom discomfort will vary greatly from one patient to another.

Symptom Screening

Patients with cancer usually do not tell healthcare professionals about symptoms they are experiencing unless they are prompted to do so; this is where symptom screening becomes an integral part of the visit to the healthcare professional. Assessment of symptoms is the initial step. The healthcare professional should engage in a discussion with the patient to help with the assessment. In addition, there are a variety of assessment tools available. A more detailed assessment can be completed based on condition and type of cancer. Factors that can affect the assessment include response shift, which occurs when a patient experiences certain symptoms for a prolonged amount of time; this can change the tolerance level or attitude towards a particular symptom. Other factors that can affect the assessment include gender, social supports available to the patient, and real or perceived level of stress. It is often a difficult job trying to complete the assessment while taking many different factors that may also affect the situation into account.

Nausea and Vomiting

Nausea and/or vomiting are common symptoms in patients with cancer. The possible etiologies are numerous and varied. One of the most common causes of nausea is the treatment modality itself, including radiation and chemotherapy. Chemotherapy itself can cause acute, delayed, or anticipatory nausea and vomiting, which means that certain issues or cues such as odors may become associated with nausea and may develop if the issue or cue is observed. Breakthrough nausea and vomiting can also occur if the treatment provided is not effective in controlling the symptoms. Radiation can cause nausea and vomiting, especially if the radiation is directed at the abdominal area, a large field of treatment is involved, or if larger doses of radiation are used. Nausea and vomiting are also commonly seen in patients in the terminal stages of disease. Many times the severity of this symptom can be intense and unrelenting, especially for cancers of the gastrointestinal tract, colon, or genitourinary cancers.

The presence of nausea and vomiting can significantly affect many aspects of a patient's life. It can interfere with activities of daily life, social situations such as visiting with family or friends, and can spoil the pleasure of favorite activities. It has an overall negative effect on the patient's quality of life. Nausea and vomiting may also interfere with planned treatment, cause dehydration, and cause toxicity of certain chemotherapy drugs such as cisplatin or cyclophosphamide if adequate fluid intake is not maintained. Nausea and vomiting are often accompanied by other symptoms such as fatigue, pain, or poor appetite and can lead to worsening of clinical status and a poor outcome.

Contributing Factors

There are a number of factors related to chemotherapy that may cause nausea and vomiting. The type of chemotherapy agent used is a large contributing factor. Chemotherapy agents are classified according to the potential for causing nausea and vomiting (without the use of anti-nausea medications), with the classification ranging from minimal risk to high risk. The dose of the drug can contribute to nausea and vomiting, as well as how often the agent is prescribed. Intravenous chemotherapy is likely to cause symptoms faster than other forms because it is directly absorbed into the body. Additionally, each individual will react differently to each chemotherapy agent. Some patients also have higher or lower thresholds than others and the extent to which they are bothered by symptoms will vary. The classification system that is used to rate whether chemotherapy is likely to cause nausea and vomiting without the use of anti-nausea medication is divided into 4 categories. The highest risk category estimates that the frequency of nausea and vomiting occurs in more than 90% of patients who are prescribed the following medications: altretamine, high-dose carmustine, cisplatin, cyclophosphamide, dacarbazine, doxorubicin, mechlorethamine, procarbazine and streptozocin. The medications that are commonly prescribed to treat nausea associated with chemotherapy include Compazine, Haldol, Xanax, Phenergan, Marinol, Zofran, Reglan, Benadryl, Emend, Anzemet, Decadron, and Kytril.

Nutritional Assessment

The risk factors for nausea and vomiting in a patient with cancer should be evaluated, such as chemotherapy, radiation therapy, or nausea or vomiting related to disease progression or from recent anesthesia. A full evaluation of current medications including prescription and over-the-counter medications should be conducted. If the nausea and vomiting issue is ongoing, information regarding timing, association with meal or food intake, or other symptoms that may be occurring such as gastroesophageal reflux should be obtained. Information regarding events at mealtime and involvement of family or other support systems should be addressed. Assessing bowel and fluid status is important to determine any possible relationship to altered status. Lastly, information regarding any practices the patient finds helpful is important.

Physical Assessment

A focused physical assessment by the physician or nurse for nausea and vomiting can provide important information for nutritional assessment and treatment. Beginning with the mouth, any signs of infection such as oral candidiasis should be noted. The abdominal region can provide information on whether distention is present, bowel sounds are heard, or if an ileus is present. It can also reveal whether any organs in the abdominal area are enlarged such as the spleen or liver. The rectal evaluation can provide information regarding bowel habits and the presence of constipation or diarrhea. If the patient is vomiting persistently, dehydration is a distinct possibility, as well as serum potassium depletion and metabolic acidosis. Close monitoring of weight should be done in order to document changes prior to each chemotherapy session.

ANTI-NAUSEA MEDICATION

The following are anti-nausea medications used to treat nausea associated with chomotherapy:

- 5HT3 receptor antagonists-- act in the gut to block the transmission of chemical signals to the vomiting center in the brain. These agents are often the first choice for anti-nausea medications because they are less expensive than other medications. Potential side effects include headache, blurred vision, and feelings of dizziness or lightheadedness. Constipation is also a possibility because this medication can slow movement in the colon. Examples of this type of agent include Zofran, Kytril, and Anzemet.
- Dopamine receptor antagonists--also known as phenothiazines; work to block vomiting impulses by binding with dopamine receptors. These agents help to relieve nausea and vomiting because they stimulate emptying of the GI tract and transit through the small bowel. Potential side effects of these medications include muscle spasms, restlessness and other types of muscle movements, sleepiness, and rash. Examples include Compazine and Haldol.
- Corticosteroids-- used for many reasons including the treatment of nausea and vomiting. Typically used in conjunction with other medications such as ondansetron or aprepitant. Potential side effects can include increased appetite, fluid retention, hyperglycemia, infection, delayed wound healing, and muscle wasting. Examples include Decadron, Medrol, and Prelone.
- Cannabinoids-- the active ingredient in marijuana (deta-9tetrahydrocannabiol or THC) binds to receptors in the brain to reduce nausea. Potential side effects include personality changes, sleepiness, changes in coordination, and a high risk of dependency. Marinol is the brand name.
- Benzodiazepines-- used in conjunction with other anti-nausea medications. These agents help reduce feelings of anxiety related to the chemotherapy experience. Potential side effects include incontinence of urine, changes in perceptual ability, and a possible sedative effect. Ativan is an example.

DIARRHEA

Diarrhea is a difficult term to define exactly but is an abnormal increase in the volume and frequency of stool output. The stools generally contain over 70% water; occur greater than 2 or 3 times per day, and have a volume of more than 300 cc. Diarrhea is a fairly common occurrence in patients receiving cancer treatment. Patients with advanced cancer have approximately a 10% chance of experiencing diarrhea. Up to 80% of patients with carcinoid tumors and more than 40% of patients who have received a bone marrow transplant will have diarrhea. Radiation therapy directed to the abdominal area may cause diarrhea in up to 50% of patients. Certain chemotherapy agents are more likely to cause diarrhea such as 5-fluorouricil, leucovorin, interferon, irinotecan, topotecan, and cisplatin. In certain cases, complications and even death can occur from untreated or severe diarrhea.

Types of diarrhea are described below:

- Osmotic diarrhea-- occurs when too much water enters the bowel, usually as a result of the ingestion of a certain type of substance such as sorbitol, magnesium-containing antacids, or lactulose. Certain types of enteral feeding formulations may also cause this. Typical stool characteristics would be a large amount of very watery stools that will resolve once the causative factor is removed.

- Malabsorptive diarrhea-- occurs when the intestines are not able to absorb nutrients due to a number of reasons, including structural defects, radiation therapy, enzyme deficiencies, or extensive surgical resections. Typical stool characteristics include large volume, very malodorous, oily, yellow stools often consistent with steatorrhea.
- Exudative diarrhea-- occurs as a result of an inflammatory process in the bowel wall related to radiation treatment or disease process such as colorectal cancer. Anemia and low serum albumin are common with this type. Stool characteristics are increased frequency to more than 6 stools per day but the volume can vary.
- Secretory diarrhea-- occurs when the small bowel is not able to absorb fluid and electrolytes due to a number of possible reasons including bacterial endotoxins, endocrine tumors such as carcinoid, gastrinoma or VIPoma, damage to the gut wall that may occur with graft vs. host disease, or short bowel syndrome. Stool characteristics are large-volume extremely watery stools of more than 1 liter per day that continue even when fasting; sodium, potassium, and fluid depletion will often occur.
- Dysmotility related diarrhea—results from changes in peristalsis due to medications such as narcotics, overuse of laxatives, or an obstruction that causes bowel distention. Stool characteristics include an increase in frequency of semi-solid to liquid stools.
- Chemotherapy-induced diarrhea-- thought to occur as a result of toxicity to the gut wall caused by chemotherapy agents. Fluoropyrimidine and topoisomerase inhibitors are the two classes most likely to cause this type. Stool characteristics are frequent watery to semi-solids stools that occur within 24 to 96 hours of receiving chemotherapy.

Obtaining a history from the patient regarding cancer-related diarrhea should include the following types of information:

- Normal bowel habits, including frequency, characteristics, amount
- Usual diet, including diet history and food frequency
- Past medical history that may be significant, such as inflammatory bowel disease or irritable bowel disease, bowel resections, prior cancer history
- Current medication use, including prescription, over-the-counter, and herbal products
- History of current cancer, including location of tumor, surgery, any metastases or involvement of other organs, and current treatment including radiation or chemotherapy
- Any interventions that have been tried with or without success
- Results of medical workup for diarrhea, which may include laboratory tests, stool cultures to check for the presence of blood, leukocytes, ova and parasites, and bacteria, and possible x-ray evaluation with or without contrast.

XEROSTOMIA

Xerostomia, also known as dry mouth, is related to a reduction in saliva production. It can be a symptom of certain types of diseases or it can be due to types of treatments. The most common cause is radiation therapy, especially in the mouth area, which is usually not reversible. Chemotherapy can also cause xerostomia. Certain chemotherapy drugs such as 5-FU, bleomycin, methotrexate, cisplatin, vinblastine, and cyclophosphamide are most likely to cause this condition. Other types of medications that can cause issues with dry mouth include antihistamines, diuretics, steroids, anticholinergics, and certain pain medications such as morphine. Dehydration can worsen xerostomia as can excessive fluid loss such as that produced by diarrhea, vomiting, or diaphoresis. Other causes include surgical excision of the salivary glands, aging, and certain immune disorders such as HIV infection and graft vs. host disease. Alcohol and tobacco use can also cause xerostomia.

Oral mucositis

Age is a risk factor for the development of oral mucositis. Children have a higher incidence of this, possibly due to an immune system that is not yet fully developed. The elderly are also at higher risk due to age-related changes in saliva production, degenerative changes, and often suboptimal condition of the mouth at the start of treatment. Overall poor oral hygiene and dentures that do not fit well are also factors. The use of alcohol and tobacco products increases the risk due to irritation. Patients who are on chronic oxygen therapy have a higher risk because the use of oxygen can cause the mucosal lining to dry out. Medications can increase the risk such as steroids or anticholinergics. Patients who have risk factors and also consume spicy, hot or very acidic foods can further increase the risk due to mucosal irritation. Overall poor nutritional status can increase the risk due to alterations in wound healing and certain deficiencies such as protein or zinc.

Chemotherapy agents

The three classes of chemotherapy agents that are most likely to cause stomatitis or mucositis are antimetabolites and DNA-interactive and tubulin-interactive agents. Specific drugs within the antimetabolite category include cytarabine, 5- fluorouracil, floxuridine, hydroxyurea, 6-mercaptopurine, methotrexate, and 6-thioguanine. The specific drugs within the DNA-metabolite category include actinomycin, amsacrine, bleomycin, daunomycin, doxorubicin, etoposide, idarubicin, mithramycin, mitoxantrone, and procarbazine HCl. Drugs within the tubulin-interactive category include docetaxel, paclitaxel, vinblastine, vincristine, and vinorelbine. Problems with mucositis can develop anywhere between 2 days and 2 weeks of treatment. The combination of medications, dosage, and administration schedule are also contributing factors. Certain drugs that may not cause mucositis or stomatitis under normal doses may cause this condition if delivered in high doses, such as cyclophosphamide.

Malignant ascites

Malignant ascites is a condition in which fluid accumulates in the peritoneal cavity and is associated with cancer but does not specifically contain cancer cells. Ten percent of all ascites cases are of the malignant type. Malignant ascites is most often associated with ovarian cancer in up to 50% of the cases, but is also associated with the following types of cancers: stomach, liver, genitourinary, breast, pancreatic, and lung cancer, as well as leukemia, lymphoma, and cancers of unknown primary origin. Initial symptoms may be nonspecific and complaints may include mild, generalized abdominal discomfort. As the condition begins to progress, decreases in food intake and fatigue can be seen. Other symptoms include weight gain, bloating, early satiety, abdominal discomfort, nausea and vomiting, changes in bowel and urinary patterns, and respiratory difficulties.

Tumor lysis syndrome

Tumor lysis syndrome is a group of metabolic changes that may occur as cancer cells quickly die in response to cancer treatment. This condition can be fatal if not identified and treated. The types of metabolic abnormalities that may be seen include hyperuricemia, hyperkalemia, hyperphosphatemia, and hypocalcemia. The metabolic alterations can lead to renal failure. Other complications that may occur include cardiac arrhythmias and cardiac arrest. Neurological changes that may be seen include changes in memory, irritability, confusion, delirium, and hallucinations. Neuromuscular complications include muscle weakness, cramps, and spasms, and in later stages, tetany and convulsions. GI complications that may be seen include nausea, vomiting, diarrhea, and abdominal cramping. Initial treatment involves hydration, administration of allopurinol to treat the hyperuricemia, and the administration of sodium bicarbonate to alkalize the urine. Correction of other electrolyte abnormalities is also imperative.

Hypercalcemia

Hypercalcemia is commonly seen in breast cancer, multiple myeloma, and squamous cell lung cancer. It may also occur to a lesser degree in squamous cell cancer of the head and neck region, leukemia, certain lymphomas, and in esophageal, renal cell, and prostate cancer. Hypercalcemia is not commonly seen in the pediatric population. Hypercalcemia that is associated with malignancy is usually due to metastases to the bone. Calcium is released into the extracellular blood as a result of osteolytic activity of the cancer cells. Other factors that contribute to the development of hypercalcemia include decreased mobility or extended bedrest, dehydration, and renal failure. If the serum calcium level rises too quickly, coma or cardiac arrest may occur. Many times the diagnosis of hypercalcemia of malignancy in patients with solid tumors may indicate a poor prognosis.

The main goal for managing hypercalcemia of malignancy is to curtail tumor growth. Many of the interventions are palliative in nature because most of the time, this condition occurs in patients who are in the advanced stages of disease. A calcium-restricted diet is not typically recommended, as this does not have a significant effect on lowering hypercalcemia and may increase the risk for developing malnutrition. Initiating weight-bearing exercise is recommended to address the immobility issue. Correction of dehydration is also recommended. Finally, there are a number of medications that may be used to help correct hypercalcemia. These include bisphosphonates, gallium nitrate, mithramycin, calcitonin, oral phosphates, and corticosteroids. The patient's current medications should also be evaluated to make sure there are no medications that may cause hypercalcemia, such as tamoxifen, lithium, thiazide diuretics, and vitamin D.

Stomatitis

Stomatitis occurs as a result of the adverse effect of chemotherapy and radiation therapy on the dynamic and rapidly dividing cells of the epithelium, causing inflammation and ulceration of the mucosal cells. As much as 40% of patients who receive chemotherapy will develop stomatitis; the incidence of this is even higher in patients undergoing bone marrow transplantation. The clinical signs of stomatitis include dry and cracked lips, bleeding, ulceration, and redness. It also affects saliva production, which can result in difficulty chewing, swallowing, and speaking. Because saliva contains many immune functions, the risk for infection is greater. Pain is typically associated with stomatitis and can significantly affect the ability to eat as well as interfere with cancer treatment.

Early and Late Dumping Syndrome

Dumping syndrome is the most common complication following a gastrectomy. This can be categorized into early or late dumping syndrome. Early refers to dumping that occurs between 15 minutes and 1 hour following a meal. Early dumping syndrome may occur as a result of the loss of the stomach reservoir. The symptoms include fast emptying of stomach contents into the small bowel, tiredness, flushing, feeling faint, sweating, headache, cramping, nausea, vomiting, or early satiety. Late dumping occurs between 1 and 3 hours following ingestion of a meal. Late dumping is thought to be caused by reactive hypoglycemia in which quick absorption of food occurs, followed by a rush of insulin. Symptoms may include those similar to hypoglycemia, including headache, flushing, diaphoresis, feelings of hunger, and inability to concentrate.

Cachexia

Primary Cachexia

Primary cachexia is part of advanced protein calorie malnutrition in which unplanned weight loss, loss of appetite and anorexia, wasting of tissue, or death can occur. Cytokines are thought to be a factor in the development of primary cachexia. Alterations in glucose metabolism are possible.

Because there is less glucose available to fuel necessary organ function, catabolism of skeletal muscle occurs for use as primary fuel, which in turn leads to depletion of skeletal muscle. There are also alterations in insulin response that will then fail to trigger appetite stimulation. Protein synthesis is reduced, partly because of reduced protein intake as well as a reduction in albumin synthesis by the liver; this in turn leads to muscle wasting and hypoalbuminemia. Loss of fat stores also occurs because of increased lipolysis and the use of fat stores for energy; this leads to weight loss, weakness, wasting, and a continuation of cachexia.

Secondary Cachexia

Secondary cachexia occurs as a result of the inability to physically ingest food or absorb nutrients. This includes mucositis related to chemotherapy or xerostomia due to radiation therapy, as well as surgery for removing tumors that may affect other surrounding organs and thus alter the ability to digest and absorb. For example, surgery for removing a tumor in the gastrointestinal (GI) tract may involve removal of part or all of an entire organ such as the stomach or intestines. Other causes include damage to the GI tract from radiation and/or chemotherapy that affect the ability of the villi to absorb appropriately. Nausea and vomiting as a result of cancer treatment can also lead to secondary cachexia. Anorexia, early satiety, taste changes, and changes in the mucosa can all lead to the development of secondary cachexia.

Psychosocial Issues

Preparing food and eating is a very social function and usually involves pleasure, feelings of security, love, and intimacy. The development of cancer cachexia changes this immensely. Many patients with cancer cachexia have lost any desire to eat and often avoid social situations that involve food. This leads to feelings of loneliness, isolation, and anxiety. It can also lead to negative feelings about oneself and a feeling of loss of self-control. The resultant weight loss that occurs continues to remind the person that cancer is present. Families and caregivers may also experience some of these feelings as they try to help the patient eat, often with poor results. This in turn can lead to feelings of failure or helplessness and can create additional stress.

Early Satiety

Early satiety is a term that means a feeling of fullness after only a few bites of food. Many patients with cancer will report this sensation even when they have a good appetite. It is a common occurrence in patients with advanced cancer. Sometimes early satiety can be due to physical obstruction such as a tumor in the esophageal or GI area, or due to a tumor pressing on the brain that sends a signal that the person is full. A decrease in GI motility and changes in gastric acid secretion can occur as a result of cytokines and can lead to the feeling of early satiety. Additionally, the enlargement of certain organs such as the spleen or liver can also cause early satiety.

Dysphagia

Dysphagia can be separated into three main types: transfer, transit, and obstructive. Transfer dysphagia occurs when there is a defect in the normal passage of food from the mouth into the pharynx. This is commonly seen in people who have had strokes. Transit dysphagia occurs when peristalsis of the esophagus is altered. Achalasia is an example of transit dysphagia and is a spasm of the ring in the esophagus that does not relax, thus interfering with the normal swallowing of food. Obstructive dysphagia occurs when there is a physical blockage in the esophagus, pharynx, or esophagogastric junction as a result of a tumor.

Psychosocial Issues

Dysphagia is a difficult symptom, as it can greatly affect quality of life in many ways. Dysphagia can prevent a person from enjoying the social aspects of eating because of pain or embarrassment. The fear of dysphagia occurring during a meal can also lead to fear and anxiety. This can negatively affect well-being and outlook on life, leading to social isolation and lowered self-esteem. Dysphagia can also lead to weight loss, which can cause further issues with the patient.

Risk Factors

Determining a patient's risk factors for dysphagia is important, as well as determining how quickly the risk factors develop and the length of time the patient has been experiencing these symptoms. Common risk factors include the location of the tumor within the area of the mouth, larynx, pharynx, or esophagus. Dysphagia can be related to the presence of the tumor itself or from obstruction from the tumor as it increases in size. Radiation therapy increases the risk for dysphagia because of the commonly seen side effect of xerostomia. Patients who have any type of infection are at risk for dysphagia because it can further weaken already compromised swallowing. Patients who are already experiencing pain upon swallowing are also at risk, as well as those who have had a tracheostomy. Occasionally, chemotherapy and/or the location of the tumor can cause neuropathy in the area of the cranial nerve. Lastly, the history of the patient can increase risk, including prior esophageal stenosis, achalasia, or stroke or the condition of teeth.

Symptoms

Common symptoms of dysphagia that can occur in any phase of swallowing include weight loss, pain, and changes in sensations when swallowing. Another symptom can be alteration in dietary consistency by the patient to accommodate dysphagia. Frequent bouts of pneumonia are also a symptom most likely related to recurrent aspiration. Symptoms that may occur in the oral or pharyngeal phase of swallowing include coughing, gagging, or choking upon swallowing a bolus, excessive production of secretions coupled with the inability to effectively swallow the secretions, drooling, and the sensation of food being stuck in the throat. In the esophageal phase, the patient may complain of feeling as if food is stuck in the chest area. The patient may also experience excessive burping or indigestion. Symptoms such as coughing or gagging from secretions or an increase in heartburn can often wake a patient at night.

Evaluation

Evaluating dysphagia involves determining if it is actually present, finding the reason for dysphagia, and planning treatment. There are a few types of tests that may be conducted. An endoscopy is typically the first test; this involves using a thin tube to view the esophagus and stomach. A biopsy is usually done during the procedure. A barium swallow is conducted by having the patient swallow barium to coat the esophagus; this image can then be viewed on x-ray to identify any abnormalities. A computed tomography (CT) scan is useful to gain additional images of the area and determine if the cancer has spread; a needle biopsy is often done in conjunction with a CT scan. A bronchoscopy may be done to view the inside of the trachea to detect the presence of cancer.

Dehydration, Fluid Volume Deficit, and Overhydration

Signs of dehydration or fluid volume deficit include dry, sticky mouth and oral area. Decreased skin turgor and loss of elasticity can indicate poor fluid status. The patient may exhibit signs of listlessness or fatigue, and may experience headache. Vital signs can also be indicative of fluid volume deficit with decreased respirations, lower blood pressure, lower temperature, and elevated heart rate. The patient is likely to experience postural hypotension. Close weight monitoring can help define fluid deficit, with 1 pound of rapid weight loss roughly equivalent to a 500-milliliter deficit. In severe cases of fluid volume deficit, changes in EKG may be seen.

The symptoms of dehydration include thirst, loss of body weight, reduced urine output, poor skin turgor, extremely dry mouth, tongue, and lips, and possibly sunken and dry eyes. Other symptoms in more severe cases of dehydration include a reduced core body temperature, tachycardia, hypotension, decreased production of saliva and tears, and delirium. Laboratory data may indicate an increase in serum sodium and albumin because the blood is more concentrated. Blood urea nitrogen increases because the glomerular filtration rate decreases due to fluid deficit. Serum creatinine and hematocrit may also be increased. Serum and urine osmolality is elevated, as well as urine-specific gravity. Symptoms of overhydration include an increase in blood pressure, shortness of breath, moist skin, weight gain, edema, and a lowered pulse rate. A pulmonary exam may reveal rhonchi, wheezes, and crackles. Altered laboratory values include a decreased serum sodium, potassium, and blood urea nitrogen. Serum and urine osmolality are decreased.

Malnutrition in Pediatric Patients

As many as 50% of the children diagnosed with cancer may have malnutrition at the time of diagnosis and as many as a third of children with cancer will develop malnutrition during treatment. The likelihood of malnutrition at the time of diagnosis will depend upon the type of cancer, location, and stage. The types of treatments used (chemotherapy, radiation, hematopoietic cell transplants) are associated with both systemic side effects such as anorexia or metabolic changes, and localized side effects such as malabsorption or obstruction. Malnutrition is a dangerous comorbidity for a child with cancer and places the child at increased risk of infection as well as a compromised immune system, poor response to treatment, and a reduced overall quality of life; it also affects growth and development. Early screening and assessment for a child with cancer are imperative.

Nutrition Screening Criteria

There are no evidence-based guidelines for nutrition screening available for pediatric cancer patients that are used universally; screening practices are now individually determined by each institution. General guidelines are available, and most screening tools will divide children into low, moderate, or high risk for malnutrition. Risk factors that can be utilized include percentage of ideal body weight, percentage of weight loss that occurred within a 1-month period, serum albumin, and assessment of the growth chart. Other risk factors or criteria for screening include type of treatment planned, reduced oral intake, and type of cancer and location such as a head, neck, or brain tumor.

Risk Factors

There are many criteria that may place a child at high nutritional risk. A serum albumin level less than 3.2 mg/dL is one risk factor; others include weight less than 90% of ideal weight and a 5% or greater weight change in one month for a child or greater than 1% for an infant. Treatments such as surgery in the GI tract, radiation therapy targeted to the GI tract or central nervous system, or bone marrow transplant also contribute. Side effects from certain treatments such as chemotherapy, especially if the side effects are GI-related, also have an impact. Another risk factor in children is consuming less than 50% of caloric requirements for greater than 3 days, as well as the use of nutrition support such as enteral or parenteral nutrition. A change of more than 2 major percentiles on the growth curve, including weight for age, stature for age, body mass index, or weight for stature, places the child at higher risk.

Cancer diagnoses that impart a high nutritional risk include Wilms' Tumor, neuroblastoma, medulloblastoma, or Non-Hodgkin's lymphoma (stages III and higher or relapsed). Solid tumors that have metastasized increase risk. Acute (AML) or chronic (CML) myelogenous leukemia that is either newly diagnosed or relapsed increases nutritional risk. Acute lymphocytic leukemia (ALL) that has a poor prognosis is also a risk factor. On the other hand, ALL with a favorable prognosis does not necessarily increase nutritional risk. Solid tumors that have not spread carry a lower nutritional risk, as well as cancer that may be in an advanced stage but is in remission during treatment.

COMPREHENSIVE NUTRITIONAL ASSESSMENT

Once a child has been identified as at moderate or high nutritional risk, a full, comprehensive nutritional assessment should be completed by a registered dietitian (RD). The information that should be reviewed includes anthropometric data such as height, weight, and head circumference (for children younger than 3 years). A full dietary history including appetite changes and usual food intake should be taken, and food allergies or intolerances should be noted. Food likes and dislikes should also be noted, along with any religious or cultural issues. Biochemical indices should be assessed, including serum albumin, pre-albumin, electrolytes, and organ function. Calorie, protein, and other nutrient requirements should be assessed and evaluated for deficiencies. Any potential food and drug interactions should be noted. Input from other disciplines such as social services or physical, occupational, or speech therapy should be noted if applicable to the overall nutritional assessment. Any language or educational barriers should be evaluated as well.

IMPORTANT TERMS

The terms are defined as follows:

- Laryngectomy-- the surgical removal of the larynx
- Pharyngolaryngectomy-- the surgical removal of the larynx and pharynx
- Tracheotomy-- the surgical placement of a hole in the trachea, usually for breathing purposes or for managing secretions. A tracheostomy refers to the actual opening
- Xerostomia-- dry mouth due to a reduced amount of saliva
- Glossectomy-- the surgical resection of all or part of the tongue
- Mandibulectomy-- surgical resection of the lower jaw
- Odynophagia-- pain with swallowing, usually in the mouth or esophagus

Nutrition Care Plan

Anorexia or Cachexia Interventions

Strategies to assist the patient in dealing with anorexia or cachexia are necessary. The patient needs to be able to determine when appetite levels are higher and capitalize on those times. Large, filling meals are not recommended. Five or six smaller meals throughout the day are often tolerated better. The diet should include food from all food groups whenever possible, and a supplemental multivitamin should be included to ensure needs are met. Fluids should be consumed aside from meals as they may promote feeling full too quickly. A support system of family and friends should be available to assist with meal preparation, especially of the patient's favorite foods. Light exercise should be incorporated daily if possible to help with appetite stimulation. The patient should self-monitor weight at home using the same scale at approximately the same time each day.

Interventions for Taste Changes

The common sense rule for dealing with taste changes is if a food tastes good, eat it and if it does not taste good, avoid it. Strong smells should be minimized. Patients who are experiencing a metallic taste should avoid using metal cookware. Glass cookware can be substituted as well as plastic utensils. Food may be better tolerated at cooler temperatures rather than at warm or hot temperatures. Examples of cold foods that may be better tolerated are ice cream, puddings, chicken, cheese, or soft salads such as egg or chicken salads. Alternative protein sources such as peanut butter, eggs, chicken, or beans should be used if the patient is avoiding meats because of taste changes. Marinades are also useful as well as trying new spices or herbs. The use of tart flavorings such as lemon or orange may improve the taste for these patients. Lastly, the use of gum or hard candies can help improve metallic taste.

Interventions for Nausea and Vomiting

Managing nausea and vomiting related to chemotherapy is an important part of the overall treatment plan. Not everyone experiences nausea and vomiting but if it does occur, the worst time is typically on the day chemotherapy is received. The symptoms can be active for up to 3 days after the treatment. There are a few dietary interventions that patients may try to help alleviate symptoms. A trial of bland foods may be helpful; foods such as dry toast or crackers, flat ginger ale, or other types of soda may be better tolerated. The use of a support person to prepare and serve meals is recommended. Foods that are served at room temperature are often better tolerated. Strong odors of foods, especially during preparation, can trigger nausea. Avoidance of fatty, greasy, spicy, or very sweet foods is often helpful; patients should avoid trying to eat favorite foods during these periods as it may cause a negative reaction to these foods in the future.

Interventions for Swallowing Difficulties

Consuming smaller, more frequent meals and snacks are helpful to get more food into the body throughout the day. Care should be taken to select high-protein, nutritious foods in order to maximize nutrient intake. Additional calories can be added by using gravies or sauces that will also help make swallowing easier. Cold and bland foods may be easier to swallow, whereas spicy and hot foods may make it more difficult to swallow. Milkshakes, yogurts, puddings, custards, and other soft, semi-liquid foods are both nutritious and easier to swallow. Any additional suggestions provided by the speech pathologist should also be introduced, and the patient should follow any additional instructions for exercises, etc., to help with swallowing function.

Interventions for Xerostomia

Ensuring adequate hydration is essential for dealing with xerostomia. The use of saliva substitutes is also helpful, as this product not only contains water but also ions, buffering agents, and other properties to help mimic the action of saliva. Saliva stimulants are also available. The act of chewing itself is a saliva-stimulating process, and choosing foods that are more difficult to chew such as raw vegetables can be especially helpful; however, many patients with head and neck cancer cannot tolerate this. The use of sugarless gum or candy is sometimes helpful, as are beverages containing citric acid; however, there is a potential for increased tooth erosion with citric acid. Proper dental care throughout this period is important to help maintain teeth and gum integrity. Rinsing the mouth with a mixture of baking soda and salt will help to buffer the oral cavity. Lips should be kept moist, with the use of lip conditioners such as Blistex to prevent additional pain or soreness.

Interventions for Mucositis and Stomatitis

One of the major interventions in the management of mucositis and stomatitis is effective and frequent oral hygiene. A minimum of every 2 to 4 hours is recommended, and if brushing is not possible due to pain, a foam swab should be used to thoroughly cleanse the area. Rinsing the mouth with solutions such as water, saline, or diluted hydrogen peroxide is necessary; over-the-counter mouthwashes are not typically recommended due to the alcohol content, which may cause drying and irritation within the oral cavity. Flossing may be skipped if it is too painful or if bleeding is likely due to low platelet counts. A topical anesthetic can be used to help with pain. Oral pain control is often required and antibiotics are often prescribed due to the risk of infection. Topical antacids such as Sucralfate are used to coat the mouth and protect the mucosa. Irritating items such as spicy or acidic foods, tobacco, and alcohol should be avoided.

Cancer-Related Diarrhea

Effects of Diet

Diet modification is one relatively easy step to take to improve symptoms of cancer-related diarrhea. One step is lowering the fat content by avoiding greasy, fried, or fatty foods or very rich desserts or sweets. Avoiding dairy products may also help to reduce or eliminate the lactose content of the diet, because the ability to digest lactose may be temporarily affected. Avoiding caffeine, alcohol, and spicy foods is also recommended, as these foods may either irritate or stimulate the bowel. Sweetened beverages should be limited as they may contribute to osmotic diarrhea in excess amounts. Foods containing sorbitol should also be avoided if possible, as too much may cause osmotic diarrhea. Insoluble fiber such as wheat bran or fresh vegetables should be limited or avoided as this may worsen diarrhea. On the other hand, adding more soluble fiber such as oats, lentils, or citrus fruits may help to improve the condition. Small, frequent meals are advised to help maximize nutrition and improve tolerance to the diet.

Effects of Medication

Certain medications may worsen cancer-related diarrhea, such as antibiotics, laxatives that work as bulking agents such as Metamucil, and magnesium-containing medications such as Mylanta or Maalox. Promotility agents such as metoclopramide or Propulsid, as well as stool softeners should be avoided in cases of diarrhea. Herbal products that should be avoided include aloe, milk thistle, cayenne, saw palmetto, and certain types of ginseng. Dietary restrictions should include the avoidance of alcohol, any caffeinated beverages such as coffee or colas, and any sweetened beverages such as soda, sweet tea, or sports drinks. High-fiber food items such as raw vegetables, dried beans and legumes, or whole grains may need to be restricted. Foods that contain a high amount of fat should be restricted, as well as very spicy foods. Finally, milk and milk products often need to be restricted during acute episodes of diarrhea.

PHARMACOLOGIC MANAGEMENT

INTRALUMINAL AGENTS: Intraluminal agents are a strategic choice for initiation of drug therapy for cancer-related diarrhea. There are two types of intraluminal agents: absorbents, such as activated charcoal, cholestyramine, or mucilloid preparations, and adsorbents, such as psyllium, kaolin, and pectate or bismuth, more commonly known as Metamucil, Kaopectate, and Pepto-Bismol. Both of these agents work to regulate diarrhea through the mechanical action of bulking up the stool and absorbing the water content of the stools. They also coat the intestinal wall to act as a barrier from irritation. Intraluminal agents are not as effective in controlling moderate to severe diarrhea. Additionally, these agents are not very pleasant-tasting and may cause further indigestion and bloating; in fact, intraluminal agents may worsen other cancer-related side effects that the patient may be experiencing.

INTESTINAL TRANSIT: Intestinal transit inhibitors include anticholinergics and opiate agonists. Anticholinergics, including atropine sulfate and scopolamine, act to reduce the amount of acid secretion in the stomach and to reduce peristalsis. These types of agents are beneficial in treating diarrhea, especially for those with excessive cramping, but can often cause unpleasant side effects such as blurry vision or excessive dryness of the mucous membranes. Opiate agonists include morphine and hydrocodone. These are more commonly prescribed and act by slowing intestinal motility, subsequently causing an increase in fluid absorption. More traditional opioids such as paregoric and codeine are often contraindicated because they may cause constipation and have a sedative effect. The most commonly prescribed synthetic opioids are loperamide (Imodium) and diphenoxylate (Lomotil). Loperamide is the more effective of the two drugs and is often better tolerated. Diphenoxylate may have some side effects associated with the central nervous system, such as nausea and vomiting, blurry vision, and dizziness; it is not for use in children under the age of 12 years.

OCTREOTIDE ACETATE: Octreotide acetate is often used as a second-line therapy for patients who were not responsive to loperamide. This drug acts to stop the secretion of gut hormones such as gastrin, serotonin, insulin, glucagon, and growth hormone, as well as to lengthen intestinal transit time and control water and electrolyte transport for patients with large-volume diarrhea. It is indicated for patients with endocrine or carcinoid tumors, and for those patients with large-volume diarrhea as a result of high-dose chemotherapy, AIDS, jejunal or ileal resection, or high output ileostomy. This drug can be given intravenously, subcutaneously, or intramuscularly. Caution should be taken in patients receiving insulin, oral hypoglycemic agents, beta blockers, calcium channel blockers, and certain diuretics, and doses may need to be adjusted. Potential side effects include pain at the insertion site, headaches, or queasiness. Long-term use may cause gallstones or sludge in the gall bladder.

INFECTIOUS DIARRHEA

Anti-diarrheal agents are not recommended for patients who are experiencing bloody diarrhea or fever, as this may be indicative of an infectious process. It would be detrimental to use these agents in such cases, as the mechanism of action is to slow the intestinal transit time and this would prevent elimination of infectious pathogens from the system. Stool cultures must first be assessed and antibiotics are typically started until the results are conclusive, especially if *Clostridioides difficile* infection is a possibility. The antibiotic usually prescribed in this case is either metronidazole or vancomycin. All patients with possible infectious diarrhea should be placed on enteric precautions to prevent the spread of the pathogen.

Advanced Cancer Patients

The goals of nutritional therapy for cancer patients undergoing active treatment are as follows: to prevent or improve malnutrition, prevent loss of lean body mass, and to help improve overall quality of life. Other goals of nutritional therapy include enhanced tolerance to cancer treatments and minimizing side effects and complications of therapy. Increasing strength and endurance, improving immune function, and the promotion of healing are also goals during active treatment. Goals for patients with advanced stage cancer are to decrease the severity of side effects and to help improve overall quality of life. Goals also include improving immune function and maintaining strength and energy level while improving overall endurance and stamina.

When planning nutrition intervention for a patient with advanced cancer, there are a number of questions that should be explored. The first is to find out if there is an advanced directive that indicates the type of nutrition support desired in various stages of treatment. Also, thought should be given as to whether the nutrition intervention will improve the quality of the patient's life, as well as the overall risks and benefits of care. Patients and their families have the right to make an informed decision about the care the patient is to receive. Benefits may include improvements in nausea, cognition, and overall comfort for both the patient and the family. Risks may include the development of new symptoms such as diarrhea, increased risk for aspiration, and increased risk for infection, and may require surgical intervention if a feeding tube is selected.

Patients living with advanced cancer can still try to maintain a reasonably healthy diet and physical activity pattern. Loss of body weight is certainly possible in many cases; however, malnutrition does not need to develop. Close attention should be paid towards addressing symptom management for those who are losing weight; consideration must be given to a trial of appetite-boosting medications such as megestrol acetate. Nutritional supplements in the form of high-calorie beverages are often utilized and enteral or parental nutrition may be used depending upon individual circumstances. Physical activity can be beneficial in many cases if the patient is strong enough; however, specific guidelines are not available for advanced cancer. Those individuals with a better nutritional status or who have maintained ideal body weight will fare better against cancer treatment. For obese individuals with advanced cancer, gradual weight reduction of approximately 2 pounds per week can be achieved with the use of a nutritionally balanced diet.

Patients Receiving Palliative Care

Patients in advanced stages of cancer begin to transition from curative care to more palliative care. This type of care is focused more on treating symptoms and maintaining or improving the patient's quality of life. Palliative care does include nutrition therapy. Nutrition intervention can be beneficial for the following types of symptoms: anorexia, early satiety, constipation, dry mouth, changes in taste, nausea, vomiting, and difficulty swallowing. When care reaches the palliative stage, food should be an enjoyable activity and not viewed solely as a means of obtaining calories or protein or of improving nutritional status. Dietary restrictions should be alleviated whenever possible. For example, a patient with advanced cancer who also has a history of heart disease does not need to follow a heart healthy diet. Some restrictions may be necessary depending upon the type and location of cancer. Nutritional care should be tailored to the individuals' tolerances and preferences, as well as overall medical status.

Height and Weight Evaluation in Children

For children less than 2 years old, height is measured while lying flat on the back, ideally using an infant stadiometer. For children older than age 2, height is measured while standing using a stadiometer. The data should be plotted on the appropriate growth chart (either birth to 2 years on the WHO chart or age 2 to 20 years on the CDC chart). For children who are not able to stand due to disability, other methods may be used such as determining supine length using a tape measure, foot, and head board. Height can also be estimated using knee height. Weight is measured using the appropriate scale for the age and size of the child and plotted on the corresponding growth chart. For children younger than age 2, an ideal body weight (IBW) can be determined using the 50th percentile on the weight for length curve. For older children, ideal body weight is determined using IBW/body mass index (BMI) for age charts.

ENERGY AND PROTEIN REQUIREMENTS

Energy requirements can vary widely based on the type of cancer, amount of stress related to infection or fever, and whether malabsorption is present. Some cancers cause hypermetabolism while others do not. The general rule of thumb for cancer patients is that patients who are less active and of normal weight should receive 25 to 30 kcal/kg. For cancer patients who are hypermetabolic in whom weight gain is the goal, 30 to 35 kcal/kg is recommended. For those patients who are experiencing malabsorption or severe stress, 35 kcal/kg or more is recommended. Obese patients are more difficult to assess, but 21 to 25 kcal/kg for maintenance is often appropriate. Protein requirements can also vary, but for those patients who do not have additional stresses such as fever, infection, or open wounds, generally 1 to 1.5 g/kg is sufficient, depending on their level of hypermetabolism. Patients with elevated needs for healing or with increased protein losses should receive 1.5 to 2.5 g/kg. Many factors may influence energy requirements in individuals with cancer. The cancer itself is a factor, although this does not automatically increase energy requirements. Metabolism can vary significantly from one individual to another and some individuals may actually be hypometabolic. Other factors that may influence energy requirements include the use of chemotherapy or radiation therapy, the presence of side effects of treatment, and the tumor burden. Also, the nutritional status of the patient as well as overall body composition also influences energy requirements. The presence of open wounds, infection, or fever also influences energy requirements.

METHODS TO DETERMINE REQUIREMENTS

Indirect calorimetry is the preferred method for determining energy requirements; however, if this is not possible, there are many predictive equations that can be used. The easiest method is to determine kcal/kg requirements; sedentary individuals who are within ideal body range may need between 25 and 30 kcal/kg. Patients with cancer who are hypermetabolic or are anabolic will need between 30 and 35 kcal/kg, as well as those for whom weight gain is the goal. Patients who are under severe stress or are experiencing malabsorption may need upwards of 35 kcal/kg. Another method for determining energy requirements is the Harris-Benedict equation in which resting energy is calculated and additional stress factors are added based on the patient's condition. Some studies suggest that this equation may overestimate energy needs as compared to indirect calorimetry. The Ireton-Jones equation is another possibility but is aimed more towards hospitalized patients; however, some studies suggest that this equation may underestimate energy requirements for individuals with cancer. Often times, clinical judgment is essential in the final determination.

INDIRECT CALORIMETRY: There are a number of ways to perform indirect calorimetry. A handheld device is available but a metabolic cart is still most commonly used. A respiratory therapist who is specially trained should perform this test. The test can be done on patients who are mechanically ventilated as well as breathing on their own. The test measures the volume of oxygen consumed and the volume of carbon dioxide produced. The respiratory quotient (RQ) is then calculated and the REE can also be calculated using a modified Weir equation. The RQ indicates which substrate is being utilized. An RQ of 0.85 is desired, as it indicates a mixed substrate oxidation. An RQ of 0.7 indicates fat oxidation and 0.8 protein oxidation. An RQ of 1.0 indicates glucose oxidation and an

RQ greater than 1.0 indicates overfeeding and lipogenesis. Indirect calorimetry is most useful in patients who are severely overweight or obese or in severely malnourished, critically ill patients with many complications or patients who are having difficulty being weaned from the ventilator.

PREDICTIVE EQUATIONS: Predictive equations such as the Harris-Benedict Equation estimate resting energy requirements and the Ireton-Jones equation predicts the estimated energy expenditure. Stress or activity factors are used to determine more complete energy estimation based on the clinical condition of the patient. Activity factors that may be used include 1 to 1.1 for a patient who is ventilated, 1.2 for those who are confined to bed, and 1.3 for patients who are able to adequately get around. Injury or stress factors may also be added. Patients with mild starvation may need a factor of 0.85 to 1.0, whereas patients with cancer who need weight maintenance may need a factor of 1.15 to 1.3. A factor of 1.5 may be used for patients who require weight gain or repletion or who are catabolic or septic.

Obese Patients

Because obese patients have a higher risk of being overfed, care must be taken when determining energy requirements. Adipose tissue is less metabolically active; thus, a lower caloric intake is often required. Indirect calorimetry is the best way to determine energy requirements; however, this is not always available. A quick rule of thumb for calculating energy needs for weight maintenance in an obese patient is 21 to 25 kcal/kg based on actual body weight. Another method is the Harris- Benedict equation using an average or adjusted weight and adding a stress factor of 1.3. The average weight used for the equation can be determined by adding the desired body weight and 50% of the excess body weight. A final method is using the Ireton-Jones equation for obesity. The use of clinical judgment is also imperative in each case.

For hospitalized patients, the Ireton-Jones equation calculates energy requirements for patients based on ventilator dependence. For ventilator-dependent patients, the equation is IJEE(v) = 1784 – 11(A) + 5(W) + 244(G) + 239 (T) + 804(B) and for spontaneously breathing patients the equation is IJEE(s) = 629 – 11(A) + 25(W) – 609(O). IJEE = kcal/day; A = age (years); W = actual weight (kg); G = gender (male = 1, female = 0); T = trauma; B = burn; O = obesity (1 if present, 0 if absent). The Mifflin-St. Jeor formula was developed using data from both obese and non-obese individuals; it has correlated fairly well with the Harris- Benedict equation and may even provide a more accurate determination. The equation for males is REE= 10W + 6.25H – 5A + 5. For females the equation is REE= 10W + 6.25H – 5A – 161. REE is resting energy expenditure, W= weight in kilograms, H= height in centimeters, and A= age in years.

Protein Metabolism and Requirements

A cancer diagnosis brings about many alterations in protein metabolism. Protein metabolism is similar to that of a trauma or septic patient. Negative nitrogen balance is commonly seen, and this can become worse as the cancer grows. Part of what causes the negative nitrogen balance is an increase in hepatic protein synthesis as well as an increase in amino acid transport. Muscle mass also decreases during cancer cachexia and additional amino acids are released from the muscles. During malnutrition, there is an overall increase in protein turnover throughout the body; there is a decrease in protein synthesis in the muscles and an increase in muscle wasting. Serum protein levels are reduced, leading to an increase in liver protein synthesis. All of this contributes to the overall net negative nitrogen balance commonly seen.

Protein requirements are often difficult to estimate in patients with cancer as they are affected by many factors. Chemotherapy and radiation therapy typically increase protein requirements. Chemotherapy can cause an increase in protein catabolism, especially in patients with advanced cancer. Additional stresses such as surgery or infection also affect protein requirements. Protein is needed in the body for tissue growth and repair as well as to maintain a healthy immune system. Insufficient protein intake causes depletion of protein in the body. Enough non-protein calories need to be consumed in order to spare protein so it is available to do its job. Additionally, enough protein must be consumed to promote protein synthesis while stopping protein turnover.

Protein requirements can be assessed using formulas that incorporate factors based on current medical condition and other disease states. These predictive equations are not as accurate as a nitrogen balance study; however, they are commonly used for this purpose. For normal protein requirements, 0.8 to 1.0 grams/kg is used. For a non-stressed, non-hypermetabolic patient with cancer, 1.0 to 1.2 grams/kg is suggested. Protein requirements can increase to 1.2 to 1.6 grams/kg for hypermetabolism, 1.5 to 2.5 grams/kg for severe stress, and 1.5 to 2.0 grams /kg following a stem cell transplant. The presence of renal and liver disease affects protein requirements, even in a patient with cancer. Requirements in the predialysis stage are approximately 0.6 to 0.8 grams/kg. For patients with cancer who are also receiving hemodialysis or peritoneal dialysis, protein requirements are 1.2 to 1.5 grams/kg. Patients with cancer and hepatic failure may need 1.0 to 1.5 grams/kg of protein. For those with end-stage liver disease and encephalopathy, requirements may decrease to 0.6 to 0.8 grams/kg. For those patients who have cirrhosis without encephalopathy, 1.0 to 1.2 grams/kg are recommended.

Nitrogen balance studies are generally the most accurate method for determining protein requirements. One method utilizes the measurement of urinary urea nitrogen (UUN) by collecting a 24-hour urine sample. The UUN is measured in grams. During the same 24-hour period, the actual protein intake is calculated, and then converted to nitrogen by dividing grams of protein by 6.25. The formula for calculating nitrogen balance is (Protein intake/6.25) – (UUN + 4). The factor of 4 is added to the UUN to take into account insensible losses that cannot be measured such as those in stool. A nitrogen balance goal of 4 to 6 grams/day is desired, as this means that the patient is receiving adequate amounts of protein. If the balance is negative, protein intake should be increased. The presence of liver or renal disease affects the validity of the study as urea production is affected.

FLUID REQUIREMENTS

Thirst is the main way to signal that the body needs hydration. Adequate fluid intake can be affected by inadequate intake, insufficient fluid being provided via tube feeding, or through vomiting or diarrhea. Overhydration is also a possibility if too much intravenous fluid is provided or if oral fluid intake is excessive. Certain medical conditions such as congestive heart failure, kidney disease, or endocrine issues may adversely affect fluid status. A general guide for estimating fluid requirements is the following: 40 mL/kg for ages 16 to 30 years, 35 mL/kg for ages 31 to 55 years, 30 mL/kg for ages 56 to 75 years, and 25 mL/kg for ages over 76 years. These are meant as maintenance requirements. Additional fluid must be provided if the patient has a fluid deficit. Another quick rule of thumb for estimating fluid requirements is 1 mL of fluid for every kilocalorie of estimated energy requirements.

IV FLUIDS

Intravenous fluids are typically used to correct a fluid volume deficit in a patient who is unable to take enough fluids orally or to provide sufficient fluid for hydration purposes. Intake and output records should be monitored closely; 500 mL of additional fluid is usually estimated to cover insensible losses. A minimum of 1 liter of fluid per day is required for proper urine production and for hydration. For patients with cancer, IV fluids can sometimes have a detrimental effect by causing edema, congestive heart failure, or respiratory failure. The main issue that arises with the administration of intravenous fluids is whether it is considered part of palliative care. Providing IV fluids to a patient with end stage cancer is complicated; thus, it should be certain that the patient has specified provision of fluids in his or her wishes.

PEDIATRIC PATIENTS

CALORIE AND PROTEIN REQUIREMENTS

There are a number of methods available for determining calorie and protein requirements for the pediatric population. The Dietary Reference Intakes (DRI) can be used to estimate requirements for normal growth and development based on age and gender. The recommended dietary allowances (RDA) are also used to provide a factor per kilogram assessment based on age of the child. Estimated energy requirement (EER) or total energy requirement (TER) is another method for calculating energy requirements; this entails the use of an equation to calculate requirements. TER can be used for children aged 3 to 19 years who are overweight. Additionally, the basal metabolic rate (BMR) can be calculated using available tables. Additional factors can be added for stress or catabolism. There are other methods available but clinical judgment is also a very important component.

There are many factors that will influence calorie and protein requirements for children with cancer. The current nutritional status is a large factor. Age and gender also affect requirements; children have a higher energy requirement in relation to their size than adults. Body composition also plays a role. Children have lower fat reserves and have higher body water content. Physical activity level also plays a role. Calorie requirements are not always elevated just because of cancer. The effects of treatment may reduce activity level and thus caloric requirements; however, requirements may actually increase because of stress or infection. The need for growth will influence calorie and protein requirements; thus, the use of growth charts should be part of standard care. Protein requirements are generally higher for children of any age with cancer due to stress and the need for tissue repair.

FAILURE TO THRIVE

Failure to thrive is a condition in which a child's weight or rate of weight gain is less than that of other children of the same age and gender. Certain criteria need to be met in order to classify a patient as having failure to thrive. These criteria include weight for stature that is less than the 5th percentile on the Centers for Disease Control and Prevention (CDC) or World Health Organization (WHO) growth charts or a change of more than 2 percentiles from the normal percentile on the growth chart. Other criteria include a current weight that is less than 80% of ideal body weight for height or a body mass index (BMI) less than the 5th percentile. Sometimes children may be small for their age but growing normally, so careful interpretation is essential. If a child is classified as having failure to thrive, a more extensive workup must be completed to determine the cause and treatment.

CATCH-UP GROWTH

Catch-up growth is an increase in the growth rate above what is considered normal and expected for the age and gender of the child. The goal of catch-up growth is to return the child to his or her normal growth curve. The ability to achieve catch-up growth is affected by the type of cancer treatment being administered such as high-dose chemotherapy. Children who are receiving intensive treatment for cancer will have a more difficult time achieving catch-up growth than those who are in recovery. The actual timing of the failure to thrive in relation to disease state, stage of growth, and duration of deficit will have a large impact on growth as well. The formula for calculating catch-up calorie requirements = RDA in kcals/kg x ideal weight for height in kg/actual weight in kg. The ideal weight for height is determined by selecting the median weight for the patient's height as seen on the CDC (or WHO) growth chart.

Fluid Requirements

The Dietary Reference Intakes published in 2004 included Adequate Intake (AI) for water. The AI were based on healthy, well-hydrated people and provided a median intake range to support normal hydration. The AI is not based on weight, however, and actual requirements especially for sick infants, children, or adolescents can vary widely. A good rule of thumb for calculating fluid requirements is using the following formulas: For a weight of 1 to 10 kg, the formula is 100 mL/kg; for a weight of 10 to 20 kg, the formula is 1000 mL + 50 mL/kg for each kg over 10 kg. For a weight greater than 20 kg, the equation is 1500 mL + 20 mL/kg for each kg over 20 kg. These equations provide an estimate based on weight for daily fluid requirements.

Vitamin and Mineral Supplements

Children of any age who are not consuming an adequate diet are at risk for inadequate intake of some vitamins and minerals. The American Academy of Pediatrics recommends considering the use of a vitamin and mineral supplement for children who are at nutritional risk. The Dietary Reference Intake (DRI) or Recommended Dietary Allowances (RDA) should be used when considering supplementation. Children who are undergoing cancer treatment are at particular risk for bone issues and may need to be considered for calcium and vitamin D supplementation. This is especially important during periods of rapid growth. For those children who are receiving multiple transfusions, caution must be taken with iron supplementation, as this may lead to iron overload.

Enteral Nutrition Support

Oral intake is often directly impacted by cancer and its treatment. There may come a time when the dietitian or physician must consider initiating enteral nutrition support. This is an option for children with a functioning GI tract. Enteral nutrition is generally safe and can help to improve malnutrition. It also helps with growth and development, which may be negatively impacted by the presence of malnutrition. It is less expensive than total parenteral nutrition and has a lower risk of dangerous side effects. Enteral nutrition can be used in the form of a nasogastric tube for up to 3 months in duration without the need for an additional procedure to place a more permanent feeding tube. If enteral nutrition is expected for more than 3 months, a gastrostomy tube may need to be considered.

There are many factors to consider when deciding whether and when to initiate enteral nutrition in a pediatric patient. The location of the tumor is very important. A tumor located in the abdominal area or GI tract may make tube placement difficult. The presence of mucositis or oral ulcers may prohibit tube placement. If the child has thrombocytopenia, there is a greater chance the child may bleed from the procedure. The platelet count should be higher than 50,000/mm^3 before a tube is placed. If the child has poor immune function, the child is at higher risk for developing infection, and this procedure should be delayed until immune function improves. The type of treatment being planned should also be considered, as some forms of high-dose chemotherapy may impair tolerance to enteral nutrition. Surgery to the GI tract or abdominal area also interferes with tolerance. Radiation therapy may also be a factor.

Parenteral Nutrition

There are certain situations in which TPN may be useful such as severe, intractable vomiting, certain types of surgery, severe and intractable diarrhea, graft-versus-host disease affecting the GI tract, prolonged ileus, and severe radiation enteritis requiring NPO status. The efficacy of TPN in pediatric oncology patients has not been well documented. Some studies have not shown an improvement in nutritional status before 28 days of treatment. It may also increase infection rate for children with cancer. PN may interfere with the transition to oral nutrition. PN has been shown to be beneficial in hematopoietic stem cell transplants by improving survival rates in children who receive PN before and after the transplant.

Patients Receiving HSCT

Energy Requirements

Energy requirements for children are typically based on age, sex, weight, and other medical issues. The recommended daily allowance (RDA) should not be used to estimate energy requirements because it will overestimate calorie needs. Energy requirements can be calculated using the basal metabolic rate (BMR). Children who are obese should utilize an adjusted ideal body weight. During the initial posttransplant period, a factor of 1.6 to 1.8 can be added to the BMR; in the maintenance phase, the factor can be decreased to 1.4 to 1.6 times the BMR. For adults, basal energy requirements can be calculated using the Harris-Benedict equation. An adjusted weight should be used for adults who weigh greater than 25% above their ideal body weight. During the immediate posttransplant phase, a stress factor of 1.5 should be used, followed by a factor of 1.3 in the maintenance phase. Higher energy requirements for both adults and children may be present for those with higher activity levels, weight loss, infection, or graft vs. host disease.

Caloric Distribution and Fluid Requirements

The caloric distribution for patients undergoing HSCT is about the same for both enteral and parenteral nutrition. Carbohydrate should be provided at 50% to 60% of total calories; this percentage may be adjusted depending upon hyperglycemia. Fat should be provided at 15% to 30% of total calories, while protein should be provided at 15% to 20%. It is imperative for patients who have undergone HSCT to receive adequate hydration due to the many nephrotoxic drugs used. Typical fluid requirements are 1 to 2 times maintenance requirements. Fluid needs are affected by increased losses from the GI tract, renal losses, skin losses, or infection. Fluid requirements for adults and children weighing over 40 kg can be calculated using a general equation of 1500 mL/m^2 of body surface area. For children less than 10 kg, 100 mL/kg is used. Requirements for children weighing 11 to 20 kg are 1000 mL + 50 mL/kg for each kg above 10 kg. For a weight of 21 to 40 kg, requirements are 1500 mL + 20 mL/kg for each kg above 20 kg.

Percutaneous Endoscopic Gastrostomy

Enteral nutrition support is often required either before or immediately after surgery to help prevent complications such as poor wound healing. A percutaneous endoscopic gastrostomy (PEG) tube is often placed before or at the time of surgery. This is common practice for patients with head and neck cancer. The PEG can be placed as a precaution if the patient is not malnourished because this type of cancer can cause multiple nutritional issues such as dysphagia or treatment side effects The placement of this type of tube usually has a low rate of complications and is well tolerated. The PEG can be used to help prevent dehydration, and is useful in patients getting ready to start chemotherapy or radiation to help prevent any interruptions in treatment due to side effects.

Colostomies and Ileostomies

The location of the ostomy has the greatest impact on nutrition. Ileostomies typically have greater fluid losses than colostomies because the colon is bypassed at the major site of fluid absorption. Stools that pass through the ileostomy are typically liquid. Patients with colostomies will also experience fluid loss, as the stool will contain a higher fluid content. Colostomies may have no real effect on stool consistency, but this may vary between patients. With an increased loss of fluid due to the ostomy, fluid and electrolyte status need to be closely monitored. For high output ostomies, supplementation with fluid, sodium, potassium, magnesium, zinc, and calcium may be needed.

Enteral or Parenteral Nutritional Support

Enteral nutrition (EN) should be considered after extensive nutritional counseling has occurred without results or after pharmacological interventions have been explored and tried with negative results. The patient should have a functioning GI tract and be at moderate or high risk for malnutrition. Enteral nutrition should also be considered for patients who may not be able to eat for at least 5 days. The use of EN may result in fewer complications from cancer treatment and may result in lower hospital costs; however, EN has not been shown to effectively improve mortality rates of these patients. Common diagnoses that may benefit from enteral nutrition include cancers of the head and neck, esophagus, and stomach or GI tract.

Parenteral nutrition (PN) is an aggressive form of nutritional support for any patient but especially for a patient with cancer. It should only be considered if enteral nutrition is not an option and if aggressive nutritional support is part of the plan for medical care. PN may be useful for patients with moderate or severe malnutrition who are undergoing cancer treatment with some response to therapy and are unable to adequately meet their nutritional needs through the oral route or through enteral nutrition. Research is being done to identify those patients who may benefit from PN therapy without harm resulting from the risks of this form of nutrition. Patients with rapidly spreading cancer who are not responding to treatment are usually not good candidates. One other concern is that the use of PN may stimulate the growth of the tumor because glucose is the preferred fuel of cancer cells.

Enteral or parenteral nutrition is appropriate when malnutrition is present in a patient undergoing treatment to fight cancer when the patient is not able to meet nutrient requirements orally. It is not appropriate to routinely use either form of specialized nutritional support in patients scheduled for major cancer-related surgery. If the patient has a moderate or higher degree of malnutrition, the risks and benefits of enteral or parenteral nutrition in the preoperative period must be carefully weighed. The occurrence of infection related to either form of specialized nutrition may actually delay the surgery, thus possibly complicating the outcome. Enteral or parenteral nutrition should not be used in every patient receiving chemotherapy. Additionally, those patients receiving radiation therapy to the head and neck, abdominal, or pelvic regions should not be routinely started on parenteral nutrition. The decision to initiate either form of nutritional support should depend upon nutritional status and ability to eat and absorb nutrients effectively.

Use in Advanced Cancer

The use of specialized nutritional support such as enteral (EN) or parenteral nutrition (PN) in patients with advanced stages of cancer has a variety of opinions. The use of PN or EN as a palliative measure in patients with terminal cancer is seldom recommended. Many health care providers have differing views on the role of EN or PN in advanced cancer. In helping to formulate a decision, the input of the patient and the patient's family should be sought, and the potential risks and benefits carefully weighed, along with the best estimation of survival. The overall goal of EN or PN is to improve quality of life; however, this may not actually be possible in patients with advanced cancer due to the potential complications of EN or PN such as infection. Some patients may actually show improvement in quality of life, however, such as those with an inoperable tumor in the GI tract. Specialized nutritional support is not generally recommended for patients in whom the estimated length of survival is less than 3 months.

Low-Lactose Diet

A low-lactose diet involves reducing or eliminating lactose-containing products from the diet. The largest group of foods containing lactose is dairy foods, including milk, cheese, cream, ice cream, yogurt, cottage cheese, and butter or margarine. This type of diet restriction involves a significant amount of label reading. Key words to be aware of include milk, non- fat milk solids, whey, lactose, margarine, or cream. Products that may be substituted include soy or rice milk or other non-dairy beverages. Commercial products are available to aid in the lactose digestive process such as Lactase enzyme supplements. The amount needed will vary between individuals and should be adjusted based on tolerance. Patients may experience deficiencies in nutrients such as calcium and vitamin D.

CANCER SURVIVORS

Many cancer survivors are at risk for developing other chronic illnesses such as heart disease or diabetes and should structure their diet accordingly to help reduce the risk. Some research has shown that reducing fat to less that 20% of total calories may reduce the risk of recurrent breast cancer. The current level of fat intake is recommended to be 20% to 35% of total calories, with less than 10% coming from saturated fat. Trans fats should be limited to less than 3% of total calories. There is some evidence that omega 3 fatty acids may also be beneficial, especially for treating cachexia. Sufficient protein intake is essential to overall health and repair of cells. The current recommendations are for a protein intake of at least 0.8 g/ kg or 10% to 35% of total calories, and should be derived from low-fat protein sources such as fish, lean meats, chicken, or low-fat dairy products. The current recommendation for carbohydrates is 45% to 65% of total calories; major sources are fruits, vegetables, whole grains, and legumes.

Nutrition Care Interventions

Dumping Syndrome

Patients experiencing dumping syndrome following GI surgery for cancer should try to eat foods that are high in protein and complex carbohydrates. Simple carbohydrates such as sugar-containing foods and fruit juices should be limited or avoided because these types of foods are hyperosmolar and may worsen dumping syndrome. Small, frequent meals and snacks should be taken throughout the day, and liquids should be consumed at least 30 minutes before or after meals. Foods that are very hot or cold should be avoided, as this contributes to dumping. Foods that contain pectin such as bananas, apples, or oatmeal help to reduce transit time and should be consumed as part of the diet if possible. Patients should eat in a relaxed atmosphere, eat slowly, chew foods thoroughly, and relax after meals to help reduce transit time.

Nutritional Intolerances and Deficiencies Following Gastrectomy

Potential intolerances following a gastrectomy include lactose and fat malabsorption. Anemia and metabolic bone disease are also possible. Nutritional deficiencies that may be seen following a gastrectomy include vitamin B12, iron, calcium, and fat soluble vitamin deficiency. Folate deficiency related to vitamin B12 deficiency is also a possibility and should be monitored. To help with fat malabsorption, a low-fat diet may be implemented or pancreatic enzyme replacement such as lipase may be prescribed. A reduced lactose diet is indicated for a patient experiencing lactose intolerance. Supplementation with appropriate vitamins and minerals may be indicated to prevent deficiencies.

Esophageal Stent

An esophageal stent is often used in patients with advanced esophageal cancer as a palliative measure. If the patient is no longer a candidate for surgery, the placement of a stent allows for the relief of dysphagia. The stent works to gradually dilate the esophagus and carries a lower long-term risk of perforation or obstruction. Following an esophageal stent placement, the diet should be altered in consistency to make it easier to swallow. All food needs to be eaten slowly and chewed thoroughly. Smaller, more frequent meals are advised. The patient should remain upright while eating and should remain that way for at least a half hour after eating. The use of Coca-Cola® may help dislodge food from the esophagus if it feels like there is something stuck there. Nutritional supplements may be necessary to help maintain or gain weight.

GVHD

There are generally 5 phases for diet progression for a patient with graft-versus-host disease (GVHD). The first phase of dietary management of gastrointestinal GVHD (Gastrointestinal graft-versus-host disease) is bowel rest, and during this phase, parenteral nutrition (PN) is used. The symptoms that may be observed include abdominal cramping, GI bleeding, watery diarrhea, low serum albumin, hypoactive or absent bowel sounds, nausea, or vomiting. Once these symptoms start to subside, an oral diet consisting mainly of liquids can be initiated. The second phase is when liquids are advanced. The liquids should be isotonic and low-residue as well as low-lactose to prevent irritating the GI tract. Typically, 2 ounces of fluid are given every 2 to 3 hours to see how it is tolerated; parenteral nutrition then continues. The third phase involves introduction of solids, which should consist of minimal lactose, low-fat, and low-fiber foods. Solid food should be introduced slowly, such as by giving small, frequent meals every 3 hours. Gastric irritants should be avoided. PN can begin to be cycled and the rate slowly decreased. Stools should be formed and abdominal cramping should be nearly gone. The next phase involves advancing solids, followed by advancement to a regular diet. As the diet advances to include more foods, PN can be cycled to overnight. As the patient reaches a full regular diet, PN can be stopped. Foods that have been restricted up to now should be added back one at a time to observe tolerance. Fat restriction is not necessary if there is no sign of malabsorption. At this point, abdominal cramping is resolved, stools are normal in consistency, the amount of transit time for the stool has returned to normal, and serum albumin has normalized.

COMPLEMENTARY THERAPIES FOR NAUSEA AND VOMITING

There are many complementary therapies for treating nausea and vomiting related to chemotherapy. Relaxation exercises such as guided imagery, hypnosis, biofeedback, breathing, and passive muscle relaxation are often helpful, especially for controlling anxiety. These types of mind-body interventions are often useful for children experiencing these symptoms. Some randomized controlled studies have shown these methods to be advantageous to patients receiving chemotherapy. Massage therapy may be beneficial as well as art or music therapy. Acupuncture has also been shown to be effective for many patients; acupressure bands are now available that apply pressure to the wrist over a point that has been identified as being effective in relieving nausea. Some herbal remedies such as the use of ginger have been effective for some patients.

TEAM MEMBERS INVOLVED IN MANAGING DYSPHAGIA

Nutritional intervention is essential for any patient experiencing ongoing dysphagia; however, it is particularly important for individuals with cancer. Aspiration must be prevented and optimizing swallowing function is necessary to maintain or improve nutritional status. In addition to the registered dietitian, other team members should include the physician, nurse, and speech pathologist. The physician should evaluate when the patient is ready to begin nutrition. The nurse provides support to the patient and assists with the transition by obtaining necessary resources for the patient. The speech pathologist should evaluate the patient and recommend the most appropriate texture and liquid consistency. The speech pathologist can also recommend oral motor exercises, which help to strengthen muscle function. Compensatory strategies are also provided by the speech pathologist to assist with swallowing boluses, as well assisting with proper positioning of the body and neck to improve swallowing. An occupational therapist is often involved and can provide any adaptive equipment necessary to aid swallowing, such as long-handled spoons or special cups.

HSCT PATIENTS

SPECIALIZED NUTRITIONAL SUPPORT

The use of HSCT (hematopoietic stem cell transplant) continues to increase as a treatment for various solid tumors and blood disorders. The side effects of the pretransplant regimen are often severe and may leave recipients with malnutrition as a result. Early nutritional intervention for patients receiving HSCT is imperative; the main goal is to try to prevent malnutrition and maintain body weight within 95% of ideal body weight. Patients should begin enteral (EN) or parenteral (PN) nutrition immediately if the possibility of prolonged inadequate intake is expected or if low serum albumin or weight loss is already present. The majority of patients receive PN. Caloric requirements for patients starting PN who have had HSCT are generally 30 to 35 kcal/kg, with at least 1.5 g/kg of protein. Careful attention must be paid to fluid allotment, as volume overload can potentially occur as a result of blood products, medications and IV fluids.

A low microbial diet is typically prescribed for patients who are recovering from HSCT. This type of diet restricts food that may have a high bacterial content, thus minimizing the risk of gastrointestinal illness related the ingestion of these foods. The degree of restriction varies widely between HSCT centers. The main focus is fruits and vegetables that have been thoroughly washed, the avoidance of foods such as unpasteurized dairy products, raw meats, or meats that have not been properly cooked, and aged cheeses and any foods that have mold present. The use of many herbal products is restricted as well due to nonstandardized production and lax regulation. Prior to discharge, the patient and/or family should be instructed on proper food handling and food safety issues to avoid possible infection. Autologous transplant patients must follow these guidelines for 3 months while allogeneic transplant patients must follow the guidelines for at least one year.

Parenteral Nutrition

The decision to initiate parenteral nutrition (PN) is typically based on the current nutritional status of a patient, whether the patient is physically able to eat and tolerate the diet sufficiently, and the presence of gastrointestinal or oral complications or side effects. Examples of this include severe nausea and vomiting or diarrhea. According to the American Society for Enteral and Parenteral Nutrition (ASPEN), patients who are expected to have inadequate nutrient intake for more than 7 to14 days should be considered for PN. Patients who are already malnourished or those with graft-vs-host disease (GVHD) or with multiorgan failure should begin aggressive PN if this is consistent with overall goals for treatment. Generally, patients with a current weight that is 95% or less than their ideal body weight are more likely to have a compromised outcome from the transplant. These patients should be considered more quickly for treatment with parenteral nutrition, especially if oral intake is inadequate.

Patients Experiencing Oral and GI Adverse Affects

Parenteral nutrition (PN) is usually the standard form of nutritional support used in patients who are recovering from HSCT and are experiencing oral and/or GI side effects from the conditioning phase. Dextrose usually contributes approximately 50% to 60% of total calories; however, this must be individualized to each patient based on glucose levels. Amino acids typically provide approximately 15% to 20% of total calories. The use of L-glutamine may be beneficial for patients who are recovering from HSCT by improving immune response, improving nitrogen balance, and lowering the length of stay. Additional research is needed. Intravenous lipids should contribute between 20% and 30% of total calories. Lipids provide both a concentrated form of energy and essential fatty acids.

Enteral Nutrition

The use of enteral nutrition has not been very successful in the early phase following hematopoietic cell transplantation (HSCT) mainly because of increases in GI dysfunction related to therapies such as chemotherapy or conditions such as thrombocytopenia or neutropenia. Often, enteral nutrition can be combined with parenteral nutrition as an alternative. Situations in which enteral nutrition should be considered would be insufficient recovery of platelets or the need for longer duration of nutritional support. Other situations include HSCT that was considered to be low risk because the donor was autologous or a sibling that was a match or a case of graft versus host disease that was considered mild based on the amount of stool output. Sometimes enteral nutrition can be utilized in patients who are receiving nonmyeloablative conditioning therapy, which is less intensive and carries a lower risk of mortality than standard myeloablative regimens.

Patient Education Regarding Cancer-Related Diarrhea

It is imperative to include the patient as well as the family or caregiver in any educational efforts related to diarrhea. Any patient receiving cancer treatment should be considered at risk for developing diarrhea at some point during treatment. Patients should be advised how to prevent diarrhea or relieve its symptoms if it develops. Patients and family should be advised as to the dangers of diarrhea and the adverse outcomes that may occur such as dehydration or fluid-electrolyte disturbances. They should also be aware of the danger signals such as excessive thirst, fever, dizziness, and disturbances in heart rhythms. Also, they should be advised when the physician should be contacted, especially if diarrhea does not respond to treatment within 12 hours. Care should be taken to ensure that elderly or debilitated patients are able to fully comprehend the information, as well as anyone for whom English is not his or her native language. The use of logs to document symptoms can be advantageous in evaluating the situation.

Ostomy

Adjusting to life with an ostomy takes time. Learning which foods can and cannot be tolerated also takes time. Patients with an ileostomy or a colostomy in the ascending colon should initially stay away from high-fiber foods following surgery. Certain foods may cause gas, increase odor, cause constipation, or may not be digested completely. The best way to explore this is to add new foods to the diet gradually. Foods that may cause an issue with gas or flatulence include beans, broccoli, cabbage, cauliflower, onions, and carbonated beverages. Foods that may not completely be digested include fibrous fruits and vegetables such as cauliflower, green beans, mushrooms, celery, peas, lettuce, raw fruits and vegetables, pineapple, and dried fruits. If odor is a problem, foods such as eggs, fish, asparagus, onions, and garlic should be avoided. Plenty of fluids should be consumed to keep hydrated.

Patients with ostomies may often have difficulty with stool consistency. Stomas that are located higher up in the GI tract are generally looser. Certain foods may also cause stools to be looser, including beans, spicy foods, prune juice, broccoli, and hot drinks. There are certain foods that can be consumed that may thicken up the stool, such as smooth peanut butter, bananas, applesauce, rice, diluted tea, or tapioca. Other foods that may be helpful include carrots, beets, potatoes, turnip, zucchini, peeled apples, and apricots. It is important to prevent constipation especially for patients with a colostomy, and some fiber should be included in the diet. For patients that are experiencing diarrhea, lower fiber foods should be selected. Some foods are not completely digested and may increase the risk for blockage of the stoma. These foods include popcorn, raw pineapple, cabbage, nuts, seeds, raisins, celery, and other types of fresh fibrous vegetables.

Whipple procedure

A jejunostomy tube is often used for feeding immediately following a Whipple procedure. The goal is for the patient to gradually work back to an oral diet. The diet will typically consist of low-fat foods (40 to 60 grams per day) and should be divided into 5 to 6 small meals and snacks. Large meals are contraindicated. The majority of liquids are usually consumed between meals and only a small amount is consumed with meals to help prevent dumping. The diet should include nutrient-dense foods and calories should be gradually increased to help regain weight if needed. Sources of concentrated sugar such as sweets or candy should be avoided. Alcohol should also be avoided. The patient should pay close attention to individual tolerance to foods and adjust the diet appropriately. Often times, a multivitamin supplement is prescribed, or if malabsorption is present, a fat-soluble vitamin supplement. Calcium may also be needed.

Food safety for cancer survivors

Cancer survivors should take any precautions necessary to prevent food-borne illness. Many times, immune status may be compromised because of leucopenia or neutropenia due to certain types of treatments. Foods that may contain high levels of harmful bacteria should be avoided such as raw fish or shellfish, meat or poultry that has not been cooked thoroughly, salad bars, unpasteurized dairy products, and raw eggs. Care should be taken to store all foods appropriately, with cold foods being stored at less than 40 °F. Good hand washing during food preparation is essential. The source of drinking water should also be verified, especially if well water is used, as this may sometimes contain higher amounts of unsafe bacteria or other impurities.

Food Safety for Pediatric Patients

Safe food practices should be followed for any person whether or not they are healthy. A child of any age with cancer needs to be particularly concerned with food safety. Patients who become immunocompromised during treatment may be at great risk if guidelines are not followed. Simple steps such as washing hands thoroughly with soap and water before eating or touching any food are very important. Other steps include avoiding foods from vendors selling on the street or from deli counters. Meat should be fully cooked and raw eggs should not be consumed. Fruits and vegetables that are able to be peeled after being thoroughly cleaned are recommended, as well as canned fruits and vegetables. Bottled water that has been bottled using reverse osmosis or distillation is preferred or tap water whose source is known and is safe. Foods should be kept at the appropriate temperature (less than 40°F or more than 140°F).

Oral Intake for Pediatric Patients

Under Age 10 Years

The use of an oral diet is the preferred route for providing nutrition to a pediatric oncology patient, but this is sometimes difficult if the child is experiencing side effects from treatment. There are many commercially available products that can be used to supplement intake. For infants, there are a wide variety of cow's milk-, soy-, and amino acid-based infant formulas that may be used to improve nutrition. Additionally, these formulas can be mixed to caloric density levels greater than 20 kcal/ounce under the supervision of a physician and registered dietitian to try to increase nutrient intake. For children between 1 and 10 years of age, standard oral formulas such as PediaSure (Ross) or Boost (Mead Johnson) can be used. Many products are available in calorically dense formulations such as Nutren 1.5 (Nestle). Elemental formulations are also available if needed such as Neocate Junior (SHS) or Peptamen Junior (Nestle).

Over Age 10 Years

Improving oral intake can be a challenge for adolescents who are experiencing side effects from either cancer or its treatment. There are many commercially prepared nutritional supplements that may be used to help improve nutrient intake. Standard formulations include formulas such Ensure (Ross) or Nutren (Nestle). High nitrogen formulations are available such as Isocal HN or Isosource HN (Novartis) or Replete (Nestle). Other choices include calorically dense formulations such as Deliver 2.0 (Novartis), Nutren 2.0 (Nestle), or TwoCal HN (Ross). Some patients may require elemental or chemically defined formulations such Peptamen (Nestle), Vital HN (Ross), Peptinex (Novartis), or Vivonex T.E.N. (Novartis). Homemade supplements are also an option in which milk or another beverage is mixed with ice cream, modular products, or flavorings to provide extra nourishment. The decision will be based on what type of supplement the patient requires as well as patient preference.

Palliative Care Patients

The Registered Dietitian (RD) should be an integral part of the team caring for a patient entering the terminal stage of illness. In palliative care, the RD will be able to understand the various symptoms the patient is experiencing and be able to provide suggestions. The RD should also be able to help manage side effects of the various types of treatments. The goal of the RD is to provide enough nutrition to help the patient maintain strength and independence. As end of life decisions begin to be addressed, the RD should continue to be involved in the care of the patient by offering support and suggestions as needed. The role of the RD is not to force more invasive forms of nutrition but to assist the patient, family, and medical staff in making decisions regarding medical nutrition therapy (MNT).

Suggestions to Improve Oral Nutrition

Helping a patient to improve oral nutrition is also helping to achieve palliative care goals, such as trying to maintain independence. Simple suggestions such as preparing the patient's favorite food or providing small, frequent meals and snacks throughout the day may be helpful. The atmosphere in which the patient eats is also important. Eating in the family dining room rather than in bed or making the bedroom as pleasing as possible to encourage oral intake are other suggestions. Looking at a bedpan is not very appetizing. The pleasure of companionship while eating is recommended. Food should never be forced, just offered. The caregiver should also remember that tastes and preferences may frequently change and that having patience is key in dealing with this situation. Any amount of activity the patient can do throughout the day helps to stimulate appetite. The use of either homemade or commercially made nutritional drinks may be an easy way to provide extra calories during the day.

Deciding Nutritional Support

Well Nourished Patients

First, the nutritional status of the patient is assessed; the decision-making process branches off from there. If the patient is well nourished, the next step is determining if the patient is meeting more than 50% of calorie and protein requirements. If the patient is meeting these requirements, the plan will be to monitor the patient closely. If the patient is not meeting requirements, the next step is to determine if the planned treatment will negatively affect nutritional status. If this is likely, then the next determination is whether the GI tract is functional and if nutritional support will be required for more than a week. If the GI tract is functional, enteral nutrition in the form of tube feeding should be planned. If it is not functional, total parenteral nutrition should be planned until the GI tract is able to tolerate enteral nutrition.

Malnourished Patients

A malnourished patient with cancer will likely require nutritional support. If the patient has had up to a 10% weight change, has an albumin level between 3.2 and 3.5 mg/dL, and is between 81% to 90% ideal body weight, further steps need to be taken. If the planned treatment will negatively affect nutritional status, it should be determined whether enteral or parental nutrition is warranted based on whether the GI tract is functioning. If the patient is severely malnourished with greater than a 10% change in weight, a current weight that is less than 80% of ideal, and a serum albumin level less than 3.2 mg/dL, more aggressive nutrition is warranted. If the GI tract is functioning, a nasogastric tube should be placed if the patient has a gag reflex. Otherwise, other options for feeding tubes should be explored. If the GI tract is not functional and the patient is expected to need nutrition for more than a week, total parenteral nutrition may be indicated.

Modular Products

There are many types of modular products available to help increase certain macronutrients required by patients with cancer. Protein modulars include Casec (Novartis), ProMod (Ross), and Beneprotein (Novartis). Non-fat dry milk powder is also easily available in the supermarket. Carbohydrate modulars include Polycose in powdered or liquid form (Ross), Moducal (Novartis), and Benecalorie (Novartis). Fat modulars include Microlipid (Novartis), MCT oil (Novartis), and vegetable oil in the form of long-chain fats; these are available in the supermarket. Another modular product available is Duocal from SHS, which combines fat and carbohydrate in a powder form. Fiber modulars are also available in the form of pectin or Benefiber (Novartis).

Enteral nutrition

Physiologic benefits

There are many benefits of enteral nutrition, especially for oncology patients. Enteral nutrition helps to prevent cholestasis of the liver because it stimulates the flow of bile. Many nutrients utilize the portal system for absorption, which in turn helps to promote protein synthesis. Enteral nutrition is also thought to reduce the likelihood of bacterial translocation, which may lead to sepsis or multisystem organ failure; this is especially dangerous for a patient with cancer. Enteral nutrition in the preoperative phase is often beneficial in improving nutritional status along with decreasing risk of morbidity and mortality. Enteral nutrition can provide a source of fiber, usually in the form of soy polysaccharides, which is important for the health of the GI tract. Other types of soluble fiber such as guar help to improve diarrhea in certain patients.

Financial and safety benefits

Enteral nutrition is also a safer choice than parenteral nutrition because it has a lower risk of infection, decreases length of stay in a hospital, and does not expose the patient to certain risks such as catheter sepsis or pneumothorax that may be associated with parenteral nutrition. Postoperative complications are also reduced when enteral nutrition is chosen over parenteral nutrition. The entire enteral nutrition process, including formulas and equipment, is less expensive than parenteral nutrition. The medical staff needed to administer enteral nutrition, such as RNs, does not require as much training as with parenteral nutrition. It is important to note that although enteral nutrition is less expensive than parenteral nutrition, if it is not covered by insurance, it will still be very costly and may cause financial hardship for some oncology patients.

General indications for adult patients

Enteral nutrition is indicated for a patient with malnutrition who is not able to sustain himself or herself nutritionally with an oral diet. The GI tract must be working properly and access for enteral nutrition must be obtained safely and relatively easily. Strong evidence exists to support the use of enteral nutrition in severely malnourished patients; such patients will reap the greatest benefits from enteral nutrition. Some research suggests that oncology patients who have lost more than 10% of their body weight obtain the greatest positive impact from enteral nutrition. The American Society for Parenteral and Enteral Nutrition (ASPEN) has developed guidelines that recommend nutritional support for oncology patients with malnutrition who are actively receiving anti-cancer therapy such as radiation or chemotherapy or for oncology patients who are receiving anti-cancer treatment but are not able to sustain an oral diet for 7 days or longer. Additionally, those patients with head and neck, pancreatic, esophageal, or gastric cancer are likely have a high indication for enteral nutrition.

Formula selection

The registered dietitian (RD) should be an integral part of the team providing nutritional care to a patient with cancer, especially in the decision to start enteral nutrition. There are many factors to consider; the first is determining if the GI tract is fully functional. Another factor to consider is overall organ function, especially liver and kidney function. A general review of laboratory data should occur in conjunction with organ function to determine if any nutrient restrictions such as protein are required. The fluid status of the patient should be considered, especially if fluid restriction is warranted. Insurance coverage is another factor; for example, it should be determined if insurance will pay for a certain formula, and if so, what type of documentation will be required by the insurance company. If the formula selected is not covered by insurance or if insurance only covers a portion of the formula, an alternative formula or plan should be considered; in this case, perhaps a less expensive formula can be used.

LONG TERM ENTERAL ACCESS AND CONTRAINDICATIONS

Patients with head and neck cancer are at high risk for malnutrition and frequently require enteral nutrition support. Patients can usually tolerate enteral nutrition delivered into the stomach or the jejunum. Feeding tubes can often be placed endoscopically; however, surgical placement is also possible depending upon the circumstances of the case. Gastrostomy tubes are sometimes used for patients getting ready to receive radiation therapy to help prevent loss of nutritional status. For patients with esophageal cancer, endoscopic or surgical placement of a gastrostomy tube is an option. Feeding tubes are sometimes advanced into the duodenum. Patients with gastric cancer most often require endoscopically or surgically placed jejunostomy tubes due to the possibility of dumping syndrome following surgery. Patients with pancreatic cancer most often require a jejunostomy tube placed surgically due to the possibility of malabsorption or gastric outlet obstruction.

ADMINISTRATION SCHEDULES

The type of administration schedule that is selected depends on the location of the feeding tube and the ability of the patient to tolerate tube feeding. Continuous infusion is one form of administration, which involves the use of an infusion pump. This type of administration is usually better tolerated because it is delivered in slower increments over a 24-hour period. Continuous infusion is recommended for patients with a jejunostomy tube. Disadvantages of continuous infusion are the need for additional equipment and the need to be connected to a pump, which may limit mobility and activity. Cycled feedings are a variation of continuous infusion but the feeding schedule is designed to be delivered over a specified period of time, such as over 10 to12 hours while the patient is sleeping. The advantage of a cycled schedule is the ability to have time off the pump in order to receive partial nutrition while improving oral nutrition. The disadvantage is equipment requirements, such as an infusion pump and tubing.

Bolus feedings may be used with feeding tubes located in the stomach. A syringe is used to administer a certain volume of formula, usually between 240 to 500 mL per feeding. The feeding is administered over a relatively short period of time, such as 20 minutes. Patients who are in rehabilitation facilities or at home are typical recipients of this type of schedule. The advantages are that there is less equipment involved than for continuous infusion, which allows for greater mobility. It also has a faster administration schedule than that of continuous or cycled feedings. The disadvantages are that tolerance may be an issue, with the potential for nausea, vomiting, diarrhea, abdominal distention, or cramping; aspiration is also a risk. Intermittent feedings deliver between 300 and 600 mL of formula over a period of 30 to 60 minutes. Gravity drip is typically used, but in some cases, an infusion pump may be utilized. Disadvantages include the chance of poor tolerance. The equipment requirements are higher for intermittent feedings than for bolus feedings.

TYPES OF FEEDING ENTEROSTOMIES

A percutaneous endoscopic gastrostomy is commonly called a PEG and is the most commonly performed procedure for obtaining enteral access. An upper endoscopy is required to help visualize the abdomen. A needle is pushed through the anterior abdominal wall into the stomach; the tube is then threaded over the needle into the stomach and secured in place. It is a less invasive procedure than other types of gastrostomies. An open gastrostomy is placed into the abdominal wall during surgery and requires the use of anesthesia. A laparoscopic gastrostomy is a tube that is placed through the abdominal wall under general anesthesia but is less invasive than an open gastrostomy. A cervical pharyngostomy is a feeding tube that is placed during surgery through the pharynx into the stomach.

An endoscopic jejunostomy placed through the gastrostomy is known as a JET-PEG or PEJ; in this procedure, a smaller tube is threaded through the existing gastrostomy tube and placed in the jejunum. These types of tubes may sometimes migrate back up into the stomach. An open jejunostomy is a procedure in which a feeding tube is placed surgically through the abdominal wall into the jejunum. A laparoscopic jejunostomy is also performed by surgical placement of a tube into the jejunum but has fewer complications than an open jejunostomy. Jejunal access is generally indicated for patients who are at high risk for aspiration or who are actively aspirating. Also, patients with gastric outlet obstruction or gastroparesis should receive this type of tube. If the tube is placed beyond the ligament of Treitz, there is a lower risk for aspiration and subsequent pneumonia. A continuous infusion is required, although the rate may be cycled if desired.

NASOENTERIC ACCESS

Nasoenteric access is a type of feeding tube inserted through the nose and typically placed into the stomach. Nasoenteric tubes may also be placed in the duodenum or jejunum. Nasoenteric tubes are indicated for patients who require enteral nutrition support for less than 4 weeks. Nasoenteric tubes are typically 8 to 12 French (Fr); these tubes are softer and more flexible, making them more comfortable for patients. Tubes may be as small as 5 Fr or as large as 14Fr as needed for medication administration or for gastric decompression. Enteral nutrition can typically start as early as 1 to 4 hours following placement. A full-strength isotonic formula can be selected and initiated at 25 mL/hour. Tube feedings can generally be increased by 10 to 20 mL/hour every 4 to 6 hours if tolerated until the goal tube feeding rate is achieved.

POLYMERIC FORMULAS

STANDARD AND HIGH NITROGEN

A polymeric formula is a formula that contains intact carbohydrates, fat, and protein and requires normal digestion and absorption abilities. The majority of polymeric formulas are both lactose- and gluten-free. The protein source is typically casein- or soy-based. Standard formulas are used for most patients who require tube feedings; these are 1.0 to 1.2 calorie/mL and are isotonic. Examples of standard formulas include Osmolite 1.0 (Ross) and Nutren (Nestle). High-nitrogen formulas are used for patients who have elevated protein needs, such as following surgery or during healing. These formulas typically provide 40 to 66 grams of protein/L, are usually 1 to 2 calorie/mL, and may be isotonic or hypertonic. Examples of high-nitrogen formulas include Nutren Replete (Nestle), Isosource HN (Nestle), and Promote (Ross).

FIBER-SUPPLEMENTED AND CONCENTRATED

Fiber-supplemented formulas contain soy polysaccharides, partially hydrolyzed guar gum, or soy fiber as their fiber source and are used to help with normal bowel function and for normalizing blood glucose levels. These formulas are usually 1 to 1.5 calorie/mL and are either isotonic or hypertonic. Examples of fiber-supplemented formulas include Jevity (Ross) or FiberSource (Nestle). Concentrated formulas are used for patients who need fluid restriction. Caloric density ranges from 1.2 to 2.0 calorie/mL. Care must be taken to ensure adequate hydration. Examples of concentrated formulas include TwoCal HN (Ross) or Nutren 2.0 (Nestle).

PEPTIDE-BASED AND ELEMENTAL FORMULAS

Peptide-based and elemental formulas are formulas that have been partially or completely broken down or hydrolyzed to make digestion and absorption easier. With peptide based formulas, proteins are broken down into peptides and carbohydrates are broken down into oligosaccharides or maltodextrin. The protein in elemental formulas is completely broken down into 100% free amino acids and the carbohydrate is usually modified corn starch or maltodextrin. Peptide-based formulas are used for patients whose GI tract is not fully functional due to chronic diarrhea, radiation enteritis, transition from parenteral nutrition, or short bowel syndrome. Elemental formulas are used for patients who have had extensive bowel resection, malabsorption, or other type of intestinal failure. Elemental formulas are hypertonic. Both peptide-based and elemental formulas tend to have lower fat content. Examples of peptide-based formulas are Peptamen (Nestle) and Vital HN (Ross); examples of elemental formulas are Vivonex (Nestle) and Optimental (Ross).

Disease-specific enteral formulas

There are many disease-specific enteral products available for patients. Specifically, there are products to help patients with diabetes such as Glucerna (Ross) or Diabetisource AC (Nestle). There are also products for liver disease such as Nutrihep (Nestle), pulmonary disease such as Nutren Pulmonary (Nestle), and renal disease such as Nutren Renal (Nestle). Products designed for patients with cancer are purported to help relieve cancer cachexia caused by the tumor and weight loss. These products, such as Pivot® 1.5 Cal (Abbott) are generally standard polymeric formulas that may contain specialized nutrients such as the omega-3 fatty acids eicosapentaenoic acid and docosahexanoic acids. These are anti-inflammatory agents and are thought to interfere with the pathways involving proinflammatory cytokines. Some products also contain arginine to help improve protein synthesis and glutamine to help preserve muscle protein. Some research has shown that weight gain may occur over a period of 3 weeks and lean body mass may increase as well. Other products such as high-nitrogen formulations may be appropriate.

Transition from enteral to oral nutrition

When a patient is ready to transition from enteral nutrition to oral, it is often beneficial to ask for an assessment by the speech-language pathologist, especially if the patient has had any type of head or neck cancer. Once the patient has been cleared to safely start oral nutrition, the type of diet recommended by the speech-language pathologist can be implemented with physician orders. A record of oral intake should be kept to try to determine progress, although typically calorie counts are difficult to obtain. As the patient approaches 50% of nutrition orally, the tube feeding can either be reduced or changed to a nocturnal schedule. The nutritional status of the patient should be taken into account when making this decision. Once the patient approaches 75% of nutrition via oral nutrition, the tube feeding can often times be discontinued. Oral nutritional supplements or between-meal snacks of high-calorie, high-protein foods can be initiated to help make up the calorie deficit.

Macrobiotic diet

A macrobiotic diet is one that is very similar to a strict vegetarian diet. The Kushi Institute advocates the macrobiotic lifestyle; it is their belief that many of the physical ailments that exist today are a result of poor nutrition and a less than wholesome lifestyle. People who wish to adhere to a macrobiotic diet need to achieve a certain balance between the foods they eat and the environment they live in; this involves the use of certain foods, special cooking methods, pots and pans, and the atmosphere in which the food is consumed. The type of cancer the patient has will dictate what is eaten. There is a potential for weight loss and for protein, calcium, vitamin B-12 and other deficiencies. To date, no solid scientific data indicate that a macrobiotic diet will cure cancer; any person who wishes to follow such a regimen will need to be closely supervised to ensure good nutritional health.

Food choices

Whole grains should make up 50% to 60% of the diet; these include whole grain brown rice, barley, and millet. Fruit that has been locally grown should be eaten a few times per week. Vegetables should make up 25% to 30% of the diet, with raw vegetables making up 33% of total vegetable intake. The remainder of the vegetables should be steamed, boiled, baked, or sautéed, but the microwave should not be used. Beans and legumes should make up 10% of the diet, and 1 to 2 cups of soup made from miso or shoyu should be eaten per day. Fish or other seafood may be eaten only a few times per week, and all meat, chicken, eggs, and dairy should be avoided. Seeds and nuts may be eaten in moderation. Products made from flour such as pasta or bread are eaten only occasionally. Tropical fruits are avoided as are any type of sweetener.

Peripheral Parenteral Nutrition

Peripheral parenteral nutrition (PPN) is used for patients who are mildly malnourished and if parental nutrition is needed for less than 7 days. A patient receiving PPN does not need to be fluid restricted, as it would be difficult to accomplish this with a peripheral line. The patient should not be allergic to intravenous lipids, as these are a necessary part of a PPN prescription. Central access is preferred if available because it provides a better chance of meeting nutrient requirements. A PPN solution has many limitations, including low osmolarity to protect the vein through which it is being administered. The dextrose concentration cannot generally exceed 10% due to the osmolarity constraints; for the same reason, protein content is also limited.

Home Parenteral Nutrition

Cancer is a very common diagnosis is this country but parenteral nutrition (PN) is not always indicated for these patients. Patients with moderate to severe malnutrition who have a GI tract that is not fully functional may be candidates for home PN. These patients should not have a poor prognosis and should be receiving active cancer treatment. Additionally, the patient should be both emotionally and medically stable. The patient or a primary caregiver should be able to learn and perform the tasks associated with providing PN in the home setting. Long-term central access is needed, and a plan should be put in place for monitoring the patient.

Immunotherapy

Immunotherapy is a fairly new cancer treatment option. It is also referred to as biological therapy or biotherapy. The basis for this treatment is to employ an individual's own immune system to fight against cancer. It can be used alone or in conjunction with other types of treatment such as chemotherapy or radiation therapy. Immunotherapy works to help the immune system differentiate between normal cells and cancerous cells in the body and to promote a strong response in order to destroy the cancer cells. There are two types of immunotherapy: active and passive. Active works to stimulate the individual's own immune system to fight the cancer, while passive uses certain components of the immune system that are made in a laboratory such as antibodies to aggressively fight the cancer. Examples of active immunotherapy are cancer vaccines such as the human papilloma virus vaccine that attack the virus that may lead to cancer.

Side Effects

Monoclonal antibodies are administered intravenously and may cause mild side effects. These side effects may include flu-type symptoms such as fever, fatigue, or weakness, as well as nausea, vomiting, and diarrhea. Anorexia and loss of appetite can be an issue. Hypotension may be seen, as well as headaches and body rashes. Certain immunotherapies may cause bone pain. Some immunotherapy drugs such as cytokines may have more serious side effects, including kidney damage, difficulty breathing, fluid accumulation in the lungs, heart attack, or increased heart rate. These drugs may also cause mental status changes or bleeding in the intestines. The severity of side effects is the reason that only patients in fairly good health are considered as candidates for cytokine administration.

Venoocclusive Disease

Venoocclusive disease (VOD) is a syndrome that may occur within 30 days following stem cell transplantation. It may be caused by the chemotherapy administered in the pretransplant phase that causes damage to the endothelial cells in the liver. It may present as elevated bilirubin levels, enlarged liver, and ascites. Certain patients may have severe liver damage that can lead to encephalopathy and death. Because one of the main features of VOD is rapid weight gain due to fluid, sodium and fluid restriction must be implemented immediately. For this reason, in patients receiving parenteral nutrition, parenteral fluids must be concentrated and the sodium removed from the solution. Diuretics are initiated and albumin may be used to help mobilize fluid. Caution must be taken with intravenous fat emulsion in patients with impaired liver function, as fat overload syndrome may occur.

Gastroparesis or Gastric Stasis

The development of gastroparesis or gastric stasis is a possibility following GI surgery. For a patient who is NPO, a tube positioned in the stomach can be used to drain stomach contents until GI motility improves. The tube can be clamped for short periods of time to see how well the patient tolerates this. If GI function has returned, clear liquids can be initiated, and then gradually advanced as tolerated to six small meals per day. The meals should consist of low-fat, low-fiber foods. The patient should have his or her head elevated above the stomach and should not lie flat immediately after eating. If the patient is receiving enteral nutrition, a standard polymeric formula can be selected; a jejunostomy tube is the best choice for tube placement. The tube is often placed during surgery. The use of prokinetic and antiemetic medications is essential and should be prescribed on a schedule instead of on an as-needed basis.

Monitoring and Evaluation

Small Bowel Resection

Patients who have undergone a major resection of the bowel or major colon resection should to be treated with total parenteral nutrition until the GI tract adapts sufficiently to tolerate a diet. Specific treatment depends on the location of the resection and length of remaining bowel, coupled with the degree of malabsorption. Resections of more than 100 cm of the terminal ileum with or without the presence of the ileocecal valve result in malabsorption of fat, vitamin B-12, and fat-soluble vitamins. Calcium, zinc, and iron should also be closely monitored for possible deficiency; there is a risk for electrolyte abnormalities. Blood glucose levels should be monitored closely. Gastroparesis may also develop.

Evaluation of Diarrhea Treatment Plan

Diarrhea is a difficult symptom to accurately assess. A decrease in the number of stools is one way to measure improvement, as well as a reduction in the liquidity of the stools. Typically, a reduction to less than 3 to 4 loose stools per day should signal an improvement. Other objective data may include the color and consistency of the stools, the presence of blood in the stool, and the timing of the diarrhea. The actual use of antidiarrheal medications should also be documented to determine if a reduction in medication usage has occurred. Subjective data that could be assessed along with the objective data include the presence of other concomitant symptoms such as nausea, vomiting, anorexia, abdominal pain, or lethargy.

Refeeding Syndrome

Any patient at risk of refeeding syndrome requires a full nutritional assessment before nutritional support is initiated. Serum sodium, potassium, phosphorus, and magnesium values should be obtained, and repletion should occur before nutritional support is started. Fluid intake should begin very slowly, and the vital signs, especially cardiac function, should be monitored closely. The initial energy provision should be assessed at approximately 50% of estimated energy needs using the patient's current weight. Nutritional support should gradually be increased to the goal rate over a 3-day period. The patient requires continued close monitoring of serum electrolytes, especially potassium, phosphorus, and magnesium. Any suboptimal levels should be immediately corrected. Blood glucose levels should also be closely monitored. Intake and output records should be carefully documented, as well as daily weights. A weight gain of more than 1 kilogram in a 7-day period should be cause for concern.

HSCT

Long-Term Consequences

There are a few long-term consequences of hematopoietic stem cell transplantation (HSCT). The first is chronic graft versus host disease (GVHD). This typically occurs after the 70th day posttransplant. It occurs most often in patients who have had a transplant from an unrelated donor who is not an exact match. To prevent this from happening, immunosuppressive drugs are given, but the best prevention is selecting a more closely HLA-matched donor. Another potential consequence is osteoporosis due to long-term use of corticosteroids that are given to help prevent chronic GVHD. Prevention entails calcium and vitamin D supplementation. Weight-bearing exercises and hormone replacement are also used, along with bisphosphonate therapy such as alendronate. Another possible consequence is alterations in growth and development, including delayed puberty or deficiency in growth hormone. Annual evaluations are warranted to monitor for any changes in growth or development.

DESIRED OUTCOMES OF PARENTAL NUTRITION

There are many potential desired outcomes for parenteral nutrition in patients who have undergone hematopoietic stem cell transplantation (HSCT). The primary goal is typically that the patient begins meeting full nutritional requirements, even if a combination of PN, oral, and enteral modalities are required. Other desired outcomes may include prevention of fatty acid deficiency or prevention of vitamin and mineral deficiencies. Maintaining stable blood glucose levels is also a desired outcome, with the goal of preventing hyper- or hypoglycemia. The goal for blood glucose levels is maintaining a level of less than 200 mg/dL and avoiding hyperglycemic symptoms. Maintaining appropriate fluid status is also a desired outcome, along with correcting any abnormal weight trends. Another outcome is to prevent any metabolic abnormalities or changes in renal, liver, or pulmonary function.

FREE WATER CONTENT OF ENTERAL FORMULATIONS

Enteral formulations can contain anywhere from 70% to 85% free water. This means that any patient who receives only enteral tube feeding as nutrition will require supplemental water to maintain hydration. Additional free water is typically provided as a flush at a certain number of times per day (such as 120 mL every 4 to 6 hours). Patients who are receiving high-nitrogen or fiber-supplemented formulations should have special attention paid to their fluid requirements to help their body process protein or fiber appropriately. Certain patients who are losing fluid such as through a decompression tube or by fever, vomiting, diarrhea, or other means, also require close monitoring of fluid status.

MECHANICAL COMPLICATIONS WITH FEEDING TUBES

There are many potential mechanical complications associated with feeding tubes. Displacement or migration is one potential complication that can lead to very serious consequences such as aspiration or peritonitis. It is essential that placement of the feeding tube is verified before any enteral nutrition is initiated or if there is any chance that the tube has been dislodged. Obstruction of the feeding tube is another potential complication. This is most often due to medications being administered incorrectly; however, obstruction may also be due to residue from the formula or insufficient flushing of the tube. To help prevent obstruction, the tube should be flushed every 4 hours with 20 mL of warm water for a continuous feeding schedule. For an intermittent schedule, the tube should be flushed before and after feedings and medications. Medications should be provided in the elixir form if available.

COMPLICATIONS WITH ENTERAL FEEDING

DIARRHEA

Diarrhea is a common complication of enteral nutrition and there are many potential causes. Diarrhea can sometimes be directly attributed to radiation of the GI tract, causing radiation enteritis. Surgery of the GI tract can lead to dumping syndrome and diarrhea. Surgery of the small bowel can cause malabsorption and subsequent diarrhea. Antibiotics are a common cause of diarrhea, as normal gut flora is also destroyed in the attempt to clear up other bacterial infections. *Clostridioides difficile* (*C. difficile*) is another potential cause of diarrhea and is related to long-term antibiotic administration. Hypoalbuminemia is another cause, along with hyperosmotic medications or sorbitol-containing medications, as these can cause an osmotic type of diarrhea. A contaminated formula may cause diarrhea, especially if the patient is immunocompromised. Lactose is rarely the cause of diarrhea because the majority of enteral formulas are lactose-free.

The first possible intervention for a patient with diarrhea receiving enteral nutrition is to assess the type of formula being provided. Sometimes a simple switch from a fiber-free formula to a fiber-containing formula is enough to make a difference. A temporary decrease in the administration rate may help, followed by a gradual increase in the rate back to goal. The patient should be reassessed for possible overfeeding and the formula adjusted accordingly. If malabsorption is the cause of diarrhea, consultation with a gastroenterologist is indicated to determine if pancreatic enzymes are necessary. For potential bacterial contamination, clean technique should always be utilized and policy should be followed for the changing of tubing and the hang time of formula. The medication schedule should be closely reviewed for antibiotics, sorbitol-containing medications, magnesium-containing antacids, potassium, or phosphorus supplements. Discussion with the physician and/or pharmacist is recommended. Antimotility agents may need to be added to help control diarrhea.

Reflux or Regurgitation

Aspiration is a potential consequence of reflux or regurgitation, especially if the patient is weakened from cancer or its treatment. Regurgitation can occur if the formula is provided too quickly and/or the patient lies down immediately after receiving large volumes of formula. Gastric residuals are typically checked using a large syringe. There is still great debate about the quantity of residuals required for tube feeding. Generally, recommendations are to hold tube feedings if the residual is greater than 500mL. Most healthcare facilities should have policies in place regarding this matter. Steps that can be taken to decrease the risk of regurgitation and aspiration include elevation of the head of the bed to 30 to 45 degrees and to prescribe a continuous feeding rather than bolus or intermittent schedule. Tube placement beyond the pyloric sphincter is also recommended. Patients who require less sedation have a lower risk of aspiration; therefore, the use of sedation should be reviewed.

Nausea and Vomiting, Abdominal Cramping, Bloating, and Constipation

Nausea, vomiting, cramping, and bloating may be due to formula being administered too quickly or at a temperature that is too low. This can be addressed by reducing the rate of the tube feeding or by allowing the formula to warm up to room temperature before administering. Another potential cause of these issues is a fat content that is too high. This can be addressed by changing to a formula that is lower in fat. Constipation can be caused by providing too little free water; this can be remedied by reassessing free water requirements and supplementing accordingly. Another cause of constipation is a decrease in GI motility or too little fiber. This can be addressed by adding a source of fiber or a using a fiber-containing formulation, providing prune juice flushes, or using a stool softener. If the patient is able to increase physical activity, this is always a good way to get bowels moving.

Medication Interactions with Enteral Formula

Phenytoin binds with enteral formulas when given at the same time, thus decreasing the serum level of phenytoin, which may lead to complications. Vitamin K can interact with warfarin, and when given at the same time as the enteral formula, may cause decreased bioavailability of warfarin, which may impact coagulation. Giving theophylline at the same time as the enteral formula decreases the absorption of theophylline, thus potentially affecting respiratory function. Antacids and H_2 blockers can change the pH of the stomach, leading to bacterial migration from the stomach to other parts of the body and increasing the risk of infection. Furosemide can cause diarrhea because it contains sorbitol. Ciprofloxacin administered at the same time as the enteral formula significantly decreases the bioavailability of the medication; thus, the patient does not receive the desired effects.

Discharge Needs for Patients with Enteral Nutrition

Discharge planning should ideally begin when the patient is admitted to the hospital and is an ongoing process. When enteral nutrition is initiated, teaching can also begin if appropriate.

Education involves the patient if he or she is motivated and able to learn, as well as any caretakers in the home setting. Education starts in the hospital and continues at home. Educational issues to address include the type of formula being provided and instruction on use of equipment such as the pump, tubing, syringes, etc. Education on use of other types of supplies such as dressings or feeding tube maintenance is indicated. Arrangements for at-home caregivers such as nurses or home health aides should be arranged in advance so they can be scheduled when the patient is discharged. Prescription insurance coverage should be fully explored with a plan in place for payment because many types of insurance, as well as Medicare and Medicaid, may only cover a portion of the expense. The patient also requires contact numbers for help with issues that may arise once at home.

Palliative and Hospice Care

Palliative care and hospice care are terms that are often used to mean the same thing. Hospice care is a program that involves taking care of the patient at the end of life, either at home, in a healthcare facility, or in a hospice facility. Palliative care is care provided to the patient near the end of their life, but death is not necessarily imminent. It is a type of care geared towards easing the symptoms the patient may be experiencing. Other objectives of palliative care are to help the patient deal with emotions such as anxiety or fear associated with having a terminal illness. Palliative care also helps a patient remain as independent for as long a period of time as possible. Services that may be offered as part of palliative care may be home nursing visits, medical equipment, enteral nutrition, and follow-up care.

Paraneoplastic Syndromes

Paraneoplastic syndromes are medical conditions that are caused by tumor secretions. These secretions include hormones and cytokines such as tumor necrosis factor or interleukin-1. Hypercalcemia present in advanced cancer such as in multiple myeloma, kidney cancer, or lung cancer is often a result of prostaglandins or osteoclast-activating factor. Hypercalcemia related to this is not usually responsive to dietary interventions such as a reduced calcium diet. Hypoglycemia in advanced cancer can sometimes be attributed to either insulin-secreting islet cell tumors or mesenchymal tumors such as carcinoids or sarcomas. SIADH is usually associated with small-cell lung cancer and should be treated with fluid restriction, intravenous saline, and diuretics.

Nutrition for Complications of Advanced Cancer

Bowel Obstruction and Steroid-Induced Hyperglycemia

Bowel obstructions are a possible complication of many different types of cancers, including ovarian, pelvic, pancreatic, and certain types of gastrointestinal cancers. Palliative care involves the implementation of a soft diet, incorporating foods that are well-cooked, very soft, and chewed thoroughly to help with prevention. Raw fruits and vegetables should be avoided, along with nuts, skins, and seeds. Acute bowel obstruction may be managed with intravenous fluids, gastric decompression, and bowel rest; parenteral nutrition is rarely indicated. Steroid-induced hyperglycemia may be managed with a diet with no concentrated sweets and no added sugar unless the patient is eating so poorly that any restriction would not be indicated. Oral hyperglycemic agents may be prescribed and are preferred over the use of insulin.

Spinal Cord Compression and Thromboembolic Events

Spinal cord compression is often due to the spread of cancer to the area of the spinal cord. Radiation therapy is often used to treat this palliatively. Nutrition issues may arise in this type of situation, such as constipation or dehydration. Constipation may be due to limited mobility or certain types of pain medications such as opiates. Dehydration may occur as a result of poor intake. Fear of the loss of bladder or bowel control related to spinal cord compression may lead to self-restriction of foods and fluids, which may lead to malnutrition and other complications such as skin breakdown. Thromboembolic events such as deep vein thrombosis or pulmonary embolism are possibilities. Anticoagulants may be prescribed; care must be taken to keep vitamin K intake consistent to keep therapeutic drug levels from fluctuating.

DECISION MAKING REGARDING ARTIFICIAL NUTRITION

The Academy of Nutrition and Dietetics believes that the registered dietitian is an integral part of the health care team and should be directly involved in the decision-making process regarding the nutritional needs and hydration requirements of the patients. Points to be considered when making this type of decision include carefully thinking about the patient's expressed wishes regarding general healthcare decisions, as this will directly impact the level of nutritional intervention. Also, the decision should not be made lightly because once the decision is made not to provide artificial nutrition, it will be very difficult to reverse. The healthcare team should consider any possible burdens associated with providing artificial nutrition and hydration and be aware that these are indeed considered medical interventions. It should be debated whether this intervention will improve the patient's overall quality of life. The proximity to death is also a factor, as initiating this intervention when the patient is close to death may actually be a burden or may even be harmful to the patient.

ADVANCED DIRECTIVE, LIVING WILL, MEDICAL POWER OF ATTORNEY, AND HEALTH CARE PROXY

An advanced directive is a legal document that outlines specific instructions regarding medical care and interventions desired by the patient if the patient becomes unable to make these decisions. A living will is part of the advanced directive and dictates the type of care that should be provided to a patient and will typically spell out what is not wanted such as artificial nutrition or assisted ventilation. The primary physician should have a record of this as well as a copy placed in the patient's permanent medical record. A medical power of attorney is a legal document that designates a certain person to make health care decisions on the patient's behalf should the patient become unable to do so. A health care proxy means essentially the same as medical power of attorney.

SCREENING TOOLS FOR RATING SYMPTOMS

The Symptom Distress Scale is a scale used to evaluate 13 different symptoms on a scale from 1 to 5, with 5 being extreme distress. It is a self-administered questionnaire that takes less than 10 minutes to complete. The responses to the 13 items are totaled, with a score above 25 indicating moderate distress and above 33 indicating severe distress. The Edmonton Symptom Assessment System (ESAS) is a tool used with patients receiving palliative care to evaluate the following nine symptoms: pain, nausea, fatigue, drowsiness, anxiety, depression, appetite, overall health, and shortness of breath. It uses a scale of 1 to 10, with 10 being the worst pain. The responses are then recorded onto a special graph and can be tracked over a period of time.

The M.D. Anderson Symptom Inventory is a tool that evaluates 13 symptoms on a scale from 0 to 10, with 0 being not present and 10 being the worst that could possibly be imagined by the patient. It also evaluates how the symptoms interfere with activities of daily life. The National Cancer Institute's Common Toxicity Scale is a scale developed as part of the Cancer Therapy Evaluation Program (CTEP). It is a tool used to evaluate a multitude of symptoms such as allergies, hearing, cardiac events, vision, pain, and gastrointestinal, and neurological symptoms. Within each category are adverse events that are rated using a scale from 0 to 5, with 0 being no adverse event and 5 being death related to the adverse event. Specific criteria are described for grades 1 through 4.

National Cancer Institute's Common Toxicity Scale

Diarrhea: Using the National Cancer Institute's Common Toxicity Scale, diarrhea can be evaluated according to the following grades: Grade 1 is an increase of less than 4 stools per day above pretreatment patterns, Grade 2 is an increase of 4 to 6 stools per day or the onset of nocturnal stooling, Grade 3 is 7 or more stools per day or the need for intravenous fluids to maintain hydration, and Grade 4 is diarrhea serious enough to cause hemodynamic instability and warrant admission to the intensive care unit. Constipation can be evaluated according to the following grades: Grade 1 requires a stool softener or changes in diet to help alleviate the problem, Grade 2 requires the use of laxatives, Grade 3 results in obstipation requiring enemas or other means to remove the stool, and Grade 4 results in an obstruction or the development of megacolon.

Anorexia and dysphagia: Using the National Cancer Institute's Common Toxicity Scale, anorexia would be evaluated according to the following grades: Grade 1 would be loss of appetite, Grade 2 would be a significant reduction in food intake by mouth, Grade 3 would require the addition of intravenous fluids, and Grade 4 would require either tube feeding or parenteral nutrition. Dysphagia would be evaluated according to the following grades: Grade 1 would be mild difficulty swallowing but ability to maintain a normal diet, Grade 2 would be difficulty swallowing requiring a texture modification to pureed or mainly liquids, Grade 3 would be severe dysphagia requiring intravenous fluids, tube feeding, or parenteral nutrition, and Grade 4 would be complete obstruction and possible perforation requiring tube feeding or parenteral nutrition. The tool also differentiates between pharyngeal or esophageal dysphagia as a result of radiation.

Laboratory Tests for Fluid Status

There are many laboratory tests that can be conducted to help evaluate fluid status. To determine urine concentration, urine specific gravity and urine osmolality are relatively simple tests to obtain. These values are increased with dehydration. A urine culture can detect the presence of a urinary tract infection. Urine chloride as well as a serum chloride can be checked, with low levels indicative of persistent vomiting and a possible metabolic alkalosis. Other serum levels that should be monitored include sodium, potassium, osmolality, and blood urea nitrogen. Elevated levels may signify dehydration or fluid volume deficit. Hyponatremia may reflect persistent nausea and vomiting.

Quality of Life with Chronic Diarrhea

There are two ways that diarrhea can affect quality of life. Physical effects include changes in hydration status and electrolyte abnormalities. Other physical effects can include malnutrition and changes in skin condition, as well as abdominal pain, generalized discomfort, and gas. It can also contribute to fatigue and sleeplessness and affect activities of daily life. Psychosocial effects include fear and anxiety related to not knowing when diarrhea will occur or what the outcome may be in terms of soiled clothing while out in public; this also causes social isolation. Other psychosocial issues include changes in relationships and degree of intimacy with a spouse or partner, changes in body image, and the ability to fully function while at work. Some patients who experience chronic diarrhea while undergoing cancer treatment may significantly change their diet in an attempt to control it, which may lead to changes in nutritional status.

Symptoms if Pain Is Not Treated Appropriately

Cancer pain can be controlled, and patients should expect all attempts to be made to manage pain. Symptoms a patient may experience if pain is not controlled include anger and depression, excessive worrying, stress, tiredness, and loneliness. Properly managed pain can result in improvements in mood and relationships with family and friends, as well as improved energy level, increasing ability to move around and be active, improved appetite and overall nutrition, and improvements in depression. There are also side effects of treating pain. Opioids and analgesics are commonly used to treat pain; these can affect the GI tract by causing constipation or nausea and can affect respiration by slowing breathing rate. Opioids can also cause confusion, interfere with thinking clearly, and cause excessive drowsiness.

Risk Reduction

Cancer Risks for the General Population

There are many factors that can influence the risk for developing cancer and many of these are controllable. Sun exposure without sunscreen is a risk factor. Smoking and any other form of tobacco is also a risk factor. The quality of diet is a large influence as is weight status, alcohol use, and activity level. There are also many environmental factors such as air pollution and exposure to radiation or certain chemicals. Screening for cancer is available to individuals in the general population who are healthy and do not have specific warning signs of a possible cancer or an increased risk of developing certain types of cancers. These types of patients require a more thorough screening on a more regular basis. General screening tests are available for many different types of cancers, including breast, skin, colon, rectal, prostate, cervical, and endometrial cancer.

Obesity as a Cancer Risk

Obesity is a risk factor for a number of cancers. Clear associations have been documented for breast cancer for postmenopausal women, as well as colon, uterine, esophageal, and kidney cancer. Obesity has also been linked to cancers of the gallbladder, pancreas, cervix, ovary, prostrate, and thyroid, as well as Hodgkin's lymphoma and multiple myeloma. Some research has shown that losing weight may lower the risk for certain types of cancer such as breast cancer. Achieving a healthy body weight should be a goal for the general population. The Body Mass Index (BMI) is typically used for assessing body weight. A BMI of greater than 29 indicates obesity and a BMI less than 25 is indicative of a healthy body weight.

Risk Factors for Cancer Types

The major risk factors are as follows:

- Breast cancer-- menstruation starting before the age of 12, delayed childbirth to after age 30 or not having any children, late menopause, family history. Age is also a risk factor. Other factors may include alcohol, body weight, and weight gain.
- Colorectal cancer-- family history, long-term use of tobacco and alcohol, and obesity. Other risk factors may include lack of physical activity, high intake of processed meats, and reduced intake of fruits and vegetables.
- Lung cancer-- the main risk factor is smoking and exposure to second-hand smoke. Radon exposure causes a smaller number of lung cancers.
- Head and neck cancers-- the use of all forms of tobacco products, alcohol, and obesity.
- Pancreatic cancer-- smoking, Type 2 diabetes, and pre-diabetes. Other risk factors may include lack of physical activity, obesity, and high intake of processed meats.

AICR Recommendations

The American Institute for Cancer Research (AICR) is a charitable organization that promotes cancer research and helps to interpret the research and provide the information to the public in a useful way. The AICR has published the following guidelines:

- Maintain body weight in a normal range (body mass index between 21 and 33) starting at a young age and avoid excessive weight gain and large changes in waist circumference throughout the years.

- Incorporate physical fitness into daily life, with a minimum of 30 minutes per day but an overall goal of 60 minutes or longer.
- Reduce consumption of sugar-sweetened beverages
- Consume more plant-based foods such as whole grains and non-starchy vegetables and fruits.
- Limit the amount of red meat to less than 11 ounce per week and limit processed meats.
- Limit alcohol to one drink per day for females and two for males.
- Limit intake of salt and processed foods
- Strive to meet nutritional requirements through a healthy diet and not through dietary supplements

American Cancer Society Risk Reduction Guidelines

The American Cancer Society has published guidelines for reducing the risk of cancer; this document is updated every 5 years to reflect new research and recommendations. The guidelines include:

- Achieving and maintaining a healthy body and avoiding excessive weight gain.
- Adults should aim for a minimum of 30 minutes per day of moderate activity at least 5 days per week, with 45 to 60 minutes being a better choice for adults. Children should aim for 60 minutes per day at least 5 days per week.
- A healthy diet should be consumed (plant-based is best) with restrictions on red meat intake. At least 5 servings per day of fruits and vegetables are recommended; whole grains are a better choice than refined or processed grains.
- Alcohol should be restricted to one drink per day for women and two for men and tobacco should be avoided.

NCI and WHO Prevention Guidelines

The National Cancer Institute (NCI) nutrition guidelines for the prevention of cancer are in line with the USDA Dietary Guidelines for Americans. The general guidelines are to reduce fat intake to 30% or less, increase fiber intake to 20 to 30 grams per day, and include a wide variety of fruits and vegetables daily. Any type of alcohol should be taken only in moderation. A healthy weight should be achieved. The use of salt-cured or pickled foods should be minimized. The World Health Organization (WHO) also has guidelines for cancer prevention. The WHO recommends elimination of all tobacco products; it also recommends a diet high in fruits and vegetables and a reduction in red meat and preserved meats, as this may have a link to cancer. Achieving a healthy body weight is also recommended, along with regular physical activity. The WHO also focuses on the reduction of infectious factors such as viral hepatitis B and C, human papilloma virus, and *Helicobacter pylori*, which have been implicated in certain cancers.

Preventing Specific Cancer Types

A diet rich in fruits and vegetables is thought to be protective against stomach cancer. Rates of stomach cancer have been decreasing over the years due to improved food safety practices such as refrigeration. Limiting foods preserved with salt is thought to help reduce risk, as well as attaining a healthy weight. In terms of prostate cancer, several studies have shown that diets containing high amounts of fruits and vegetables and fish may help to reduce the risk. Antioxidants such as selenium and vitamin E may also be useful. Lycopene may also lower the risk. Reducing the risk for endometrial cancer includes weight loss and increasing physical activity, as well increasing fiber intake and reducing fat intake. Increasing fruits and vegetable intake, as well as increasing fluid intake, may have a positive effect on reducing the risk for bladder cancer.

AICR Position on Breastfeeding and for Cancer Survivors

The American Institute for Cancer Research (AICR) has a public health goal to promote an increased commitment to exclusively breastfeed for a minimum of 6 months. Breastfeeding has many benefits, but from a cancer perspective, breastfeeding provides cancer protection for both the mother and the baby. It is especially important for women who live in parts of the world that are impoverished and without access to a safe water supply. The AICR has also provided guidelines to cancer survivors to recommend that nutritional care be provided by a professional that has been specially trained in oncological nutrition. Cancer survivors are considered to be patients who have a current cancer diagnosis and are undergoing treatment and those who have recovered from the disease. The guidelines for cancer prevention should be followed, especially by those who have recovered from cancer.

Nutritional Strategies Following Treatment

The majority of side effects related to cancer treatment and nutrition will subside after treatment stops. Some may take some time, such as return of full appetite or complete improvement in swallowing. There is no one recommended diet that will keep cancer from returning; however, the nutritional plan should be to regain weight if needed, as well as strength and overall nutritional status, with a goal of improved health for the long term. An ideal weight for height should be achieved and maintained. A balanced diet should be consumed, with foods selected from all food groups. The American Cancer Society recommends that 5 to 7 servings of fruits and vegetables be consumed, including dark green and yellow types. High-fiber foods such as whole grain cereals and breads, legumes, and beans are better choices. A diet that is lower in fat is also recommended. Processed, cured, smoked, and pickled foods should be avoided. Alcohol should be limited.

Natural Carcinogens in Food

Our food supply has the potential to contain many, many forms of carcinogens. It is not possible to consume a diet totally free from carcinogens but there are steps one can take to reduce consumption. Some carcinogens are naturally occurring such as aflatoxins found in peanuts, tannins found in grains and grapes, and benzopyrenes, which are formed when meat or fish are smoked. There are also naturally occurring metabolites derived from such plants as pepper, citrus oils, celery, parsley, mustard, or figs. One would have to consume a large amount of these metabolites in a concentrated form to raise the risk for cancer; thus, it is unlikely that an individual would consistently consume amounts high enough to cause cancer.

Simple steps may be taken to reduce the overall presence of potential carcinogens in our diet. The selection of locally grown produce that is in-season is one step. Any fresh produce should be washed thoroughly and the outer leaves should be removed and discarded. Proper food storage should be observed, such as keeping food at appropriate temperatures, to not only help preserve the nutrient content, but also slow the growth of fungus. Certain types of fungus may be carcinogenic. The choice of cooking method can also reduce potential carcinogens. For example, baking or broiling meats and reducing the use of grilling methods in which the flames come in contact with the food are helpful. Also, cooking meats, poultry, and other protein-containing foods at reduced temperatures helps reduce the amount of heterocyclic amines that are produced during broiling or grilling.

Role of Certain Foods in Cancer Prevention

Hot peppers contain a phytochemical called capsaicin as well as vitamin C that are thought to promote both antioxidant activity and act as cancer inhibitors. Hot peppers are thought to be protective against skin and stomach cancers, mainly because when cancer cells are exposed to capsaicin, the cells die. Garlic and onions, known as allium vegetables, contain significant amounts of organosulfur compounds, along with soluble and insoluble fiber, that have antioxidant and anticancer properties. Some studies have shown that people who consume higher amounts of garlic may have a lower risk of developing stomach, prostate, skin, esophageal, and colorectal cancers. Cruciferous vegetables such broccoli, cauliflower, and cabbage are thought to have anti-cancer properties because of phytochemicals such as indoles, sulforaphane, and isothiocyanate. These vegetables also contain folate, vitamins A and C, and insoluble fiber, which also contribute to their anti-cancer properties. This type of vegetable is thought to lower the risk for colon, bladder, prostate, breast, and lung cancers.

Citrus fruits contain the phytochemicals terpene, coumarin, and flavonoids, as well as vitamin C, folate, and soluble fiber. These nutrients are thought to inhibit cancer and have antioxidant properties, as well as to stimulate anticancer enzymes. They are thought to protect against mouth, stomach, and esophageal cancers. Tomatoes and red grapefruit contain lycopene, as well as vitamin C and soluble fiber. The antioxidant activity is thought to help protect against prostate, lung, and stomach cancers. Lycopene may also help to protect against breast, cervical, pancreatic, colorectal, esophageal, and oral cancers. Fruits such as strawberries, grapes, and other berries contain the phytochemical ellagic acid, as well as vitamins E and C and beta carotene. These are thought to promote antioxidant activity, inhibit cancer, and stimulate anticancer enzymes. These fruits are thought to protect against colon, breast, prostate, and oral cancers.

Green tea contains polyphenol, which is believed to have antioxidant properties. Green tea is thought to contain substances that block the production of certain enzymes required for cancer cells to grow and stop the flow of oxygen to these cells. Green tea is also thought to have a protective effect against potential carcinogens in the diet by preventing mutation. It is thought to reduce the risk of prostate, stomach, and esophageal cancer. People in Japan who consume green tea daily have a lower incidence of stomach, liver, breast, pancreatic, lung, skin, and esophageal cancer. It is not entirely clear how much green tea should be consumed to obtain effective cancer protection; however, in East Asia, where a lower incidence of certain cancers is found, an average of three cups per day is consumed. Research continues to evaluate green tea as well as other lifestyle factors that may influence this lower cancer incidence.

Alcohol, Aspartame, Saccharin, and Calcium

Alcohol has been linked to the development of many different types of cancers, including head and neck, liver, breast, and colon. In patients who already have cancer, it may increase the risk for a new cancer developing at the same site. Also, if the person smokes in addition to drinking alcohol, the risk for developing cancer is even more pronounced. Aspartame has been linked in the past to cancer, but research has not shown any definitive link. Saccharin has also been linked in the past to cancer but is no longer on the list of known human carcinogens. The information on calcium is conflicting. Some studies have shown that increasing calcium intake may be protective against colon cancer. Other studies have shown that taking calcium supplements to increase calcium intake higher than recommended amounts may increase the risk of developing prostate cancer.

Coffee, Soy Products, and Processed Meats

Coffee does not appear to be a risk factor for the development of cancer, although it may negatively affect women with fibrocystic breast disease. Soy products contain phytoestrogens that may mimic estrogen activity and should be limited in women with breast cancer. There has been no definitive link to cancer, but it may be possible for these products to increase the risk for estrogen-responsive cancers such as breast or endometrial cancer; thus, more research is needed. Processed meats may increase the risk for developing certain cancers because of the exposure to nitrates and other processing methods. Additionally, it is thought that cooking any type of meat at extremely high temperatures such as frying or grilling may cause the formation of potentially cancerous agents. Other forms of cooking such as braising, stewing, or baking may be safer.

MyPlate

The USDA's Food Pyramid was heavily criticized for being vague and confusing, and in 2011 it was replaced with MyPlate. MyPlate is much easier to understand, as it consists of a picture of a dinner plate divided into four sections, visually illustrating how our daily diet should be distributed among the various food groups. Vegetables and grains each take up 30% of the plate, while fruits and proteins each constitute 20% of the plate. There is also a representation of a cup, marked Dairy, alongside the plate. The idea behind MyPlate is that it's much easier for people to grasp the idea that half of a meal should consist of fruits and vegetables than it is for them to understand serving sizes for all the different kinds of foods they eat on a regular basis.

Barriers to Healthier Lifestyles

The average person may encounter many obstacles when trying to adopt a healthier lifestyle in terms of physical activity and diet. Longer work days contribute to difficulties because time at home to prepare healthier meals is limited, and many people resort to fast food or convenience foods. Additionally, there has been a trend towards increasing portion sizes at all types of restaurants, making it more difficult to limit portion sizes. Longer work days also lead to a reduced amount of time for exercise and relaxing activities. Many forms of transportation such as cars, trains, and buses are readily available, making the need to walk for necessity almost obsolete. Many people also live in areas that are not conducive to walking, such as those with high crime, lack of sidewalks, or other safety issues. The prevalence of smoking in many areas of the country is also a contributing factor; this also sends the wrong message to children who observe these adults smoking.

Physical Activity for Cancer Survivors

Consultation with an exercise specialist is often recommended to help cancer survivors get back on their feet and begin exercising. Certain issues may need to be addressed before implementing a program. If anemia is an issue, exercise should be delayed until the condition is corrected in order to maximize oxygen efficiency. Cancer survivors who are immunocompromised should stay away from public gyms due to the risk of many different types of infections. Those who have had a bone marrow transplant should abstain for at least a year following transplant. Cancer survivors who are receiving radiation therapy are advised to avoid chlorinated pools because this may cause skin irritation; in those with indwelling ports, microbial contamination is possible. Cancer survivors who were not very active prediagnosis should gradually ease into an exercise routine. Overall, exercise, if conducted appropriately and under supervision, can increase quality of life.

Pediatric Cancer

Approximately 10,400 children below age 15 years were diagnosed with some form of cancer in 2007. Although this number appears to be high and is the leading cause of death by any one disease, the incidence is relatively low for the pediatric population. Typically, more children will die from motor vehicle accidents, drowning, or severe burns. The most common types of cancers in children are leukemia and central nervous system cancers such as retinoblastoma, meningioma, or medulloblastoma. The most common type of leukemia is acute lymphocytic leukemia (ALL). Lymphoma is also common, including Hodgkin's and non- Hodgkin's lymphomas. There are uncommon cancers that are predominantly seen in the pediatric or adolescent population, including neuroblastoma and Wilms' Tumor (nephroblastoma), which tends to be seen in younger children. Bone tumors such as Ewing's sarcoma or osteosarcoma or soft tissue tumors such as rhabdomyosarcoma tend to be seen in the adolescent years.

CAM for Pediatric Patients

Western medicine remains the standard of care for treating a child with cancer. Many parents want to turn to complementary and alternative medicine (CAM) as an additional therapy for their child; however, careful consideration should be given before this step is taken. CAM can sometimes interfere with the current treatment plan. The child's physician should be actively involved in this decision. The therapy being considered should be thoroughly researched using reputable internet sources and the library for scientific journals, books, or other information. Many large university-based medical centers will provide access to patients and their families to review medical journals that contain controlled clinical studies dealing with the therapy. Parents should take caution if the therapy is not based on sound scientific principles or theories, if the treatment is supposed to cure the child, is not widely and universally available, or requires international travel to obtain, or if the treatment discourages standard medical care.

Colorectal Cancer

The signs and symptoms of colorectal cancer are rectal bleeding, pain in the lower abdominal region, cramping, or alterations in bowel function. There are many risk factors for colorectal cancer, including age over 50 years, a prior history or a family history of polyps or of colorectal cancer, and a history of inflammatory bowel disease (IBD). Modifiable risk factors include alcohol use, a diet that is high in saturated fat, increased intake of red meat, reduced intake of fruits and vegetables, smoking, and lack of physical exercise. Some of the screening tests available for colorectal cancer include the fecal occult blood test, sigmoidoscopy, colonoscopy, double contrast barium enema, or digital rectal exam. The United States Preventive Services Task Force (USPSTF) recommends that yearly screening begin at the age of 50 years until the age of 75 years.

Phytochemicals and Breast Cancer

Phytochemicals are chemical compounds that occur naturally in plants and may play a role in disease prevention. An example of a phytochemical would be lycopene found in tomatoes, which has a protective effect against certain types of cancer such as prostate cancer. Another type of phytochemical is phytoestrogen, such as the isoflavones found in soy. Researchers are trying to determine the exact effect of phytoestrogens and their role in breast cancer. There is evidence that soy is beneficial to overall health, such as lowering LDL cholesterol or helping with hot flashes experienced during menopause. It is believed that soy products taken over the course of a lifetime are the most beneficial. It is recommended that too many soy products not be consumed by postmenopausal women because the phytoestrogens may copy natural estrogen, which may be a risk factor for breast cancer. For women who already have breast cancer and have estrogen-receptor-positive tumors, soy may not be a good idea, especially for those taking tamoxifen. Research is still inconclusive.

How to Overcome Test Anxiety

Just the thought of taking a test is enough to make most people a little nervous. A test is an important event that can have a long-term impact on your future, so it's important to take it seriously and it's natural to feel anxious about performing well. But just because anxiety is normal, that doesn't mean that it's helpful in test taking, or that you should simply accept it as part of your life. Anxiety can have a variety of effects. These effects can be mild, like making you feel slightly nervous, or severe, like blocking your ability to focus or remember even a simple detail.

If you experience test anxiety—whether severe or mild—it's important to know how to beat it. To discover this, first you need to understand what causes test anxiety.

Causes of Test Anxiety

While we often think of anxiety as an uncontrollable emotional state, it can actually be caused by simple, practical things. One of the most common causes of test anxiety is that a person does not feel adequately prepared for their test. This feeling can be the result of many different issues such as poor study habits or lack of organization, but the most common culprit is time management. Starting to study too late, failing to organize your study time to cover all of the material, or being distracted while you study will mean that you're not well prepared for the test. This may lead to cramming the night before, which will cause you to be physically and mentally exhausted for the test. Poor time management also contributes to feelings of stress, fear, and hopelessness as you realize you are not well prepared but don't know what to do about it.

Other times, test anxiety is not related to your preparation for the test but comes from unresolved fear. This may be a past failure on a test, or poor performance on tests in general. It may come from comparing yourself to others who seem to be performing better or from the stress of living up to expectations. Anxiety may be driven by fears of the future—how failure on this test would affect your educational and career goals. These fears are often completely irrational, but they can still negatively impact your test performance.

Elements of Test Anxiety

As mentioned earlier, test anxiety is considered to be an emotional state, but it has physical and mental components as well. Sometimes you may not even realize that you are suffering from test anxiety until you notice the physical symptoms. These can include trembling hands, rapid heartbeat, sweating, nausea, and tense muscles. Extreme anxiety may lead to fainting or vomiting. Obviously, any of these symptoms can have a negative impact on testing. It is important to recognize them as soon as they begin to occur so that you can address the problem before it damages your performance.

The mental components of test anxiety include trouble focusing and inability to remember learned information. During a test, your mind is on high alert, which can help you recall information and stay focused for an extended period of time. However, anxiety interferes with your mind's natural processes, causing you to blank out, even on the questions you know well. The strain of testing during anxiety makes it difficult to stay focused, especially on a test that may take several hours. Extreme anxiety can take a huge mental toll, making it difficult not only to recall test information but even to understand the test questions or pull your thoughts together.

Effects of Test Anxiety

Test anxiety is like a disease—if left untreated, it will get progressively worse. Anxiety leads to poor performance, and this reinforces the feelings of fear and failure, which in turn lead to poor performances on subsequent tests. It can grow from a mild nervousness to a crippling condition. If allowed to progress, test anxiety can have a big impact on your schooling, and consequently on your future.

Test anxiety can spread to other parts of your life. Anxiety on tests can become anxiety in any stressful situation, and blanking on a test can turn into panicking in a job situation. But fortunately, you don't have to let anxiety rule your testing and determine your grades. There are a number of relatively simple steps you can take to move past anxiety and function normally on a test and in the rest of life.

Physical Steps for Beating Test Anxiety

While test anxiety is a serious problem, the good news is that it can be overcome. It doesn't have to control your ability to think and remember information. While it may take time, you can begin taking steps today to beat anxiety.

Just as your first hint that you may be struggling with anxiety comes from the physical symptoms, the first step to treating it is also physical. Rest is crucial for having a clear, strong mind. If you are tired, it is much easier to give in to anxiety. But if you establish good sleep habits, your body and mind will be ready to perform optimally, without the strain of exhaustion. Additionally, sleeping well helps you to retain information better, so you're more likely to recall the answers when you see the test questions.

Getting good sleep means more than going to bed on time. It's important to allow your brain time to relax. Take study breaks from time to time so it doesn't get overworked, and don't study right before bed. Take time to rest your mind before trying to rest your body, or you may find it difficult to fall asleep.

Along with sleep, other aspects of physical health are important in preparing for a test. Good nutrition is vital for good brain function. Sugary foods and drinks may give a burst of energy but this burst is followed by a crash, both physically and emotionally. Instead, fuel your body with protein and vitamin-rich foods.

Also, drink plenty of water. Dehydration can lead to headaches and exhaustion, especially if your brain is already under stress from the rigors of the test. Particularly if your test is a long one, drink water during the breaks. And if possible, take an energy-boosting snack to eat between sections.

Along with sleep and diet, a third important part of physical health is exercise. Maintaining a steady workout schedule is helpful, but even taking 5-minute study breaks to walk can help get your blood pumping faster and clear your head. Exercise also releases endorphins, which contribute to a positive feeling and can help combat test anxiety.

When you nurture your physical health, you are also contributing to your mental health. If your body is healthy, your mind is much more likely to be healthy as well. So take time to rest, nourish your body with healthy food and water, and get moving as much as possible. Taking these physical steps will make you stronger and more able to take the mental steps necessary to overcome test anxiety.

Mental Steps for Beating Test Anxiety

Working on the mental side of test anxiety can be more challenging, but as with the physical side, there are clear steps you can take to overcome it. As mentioned earlier, test anxiety often stems from lack of preparation, so the obvious solution is to prepare for the test. Effective studying may be the most important weapon you have for beating test anxiety, but you can and should employ several other mental tools to combat fear.

First, boost your confidence by reminding yourself of past success—tests or projects that you aced. If you're putting as much effort into preparing for this test as you did for those, there's no reason you should expect to fail here. Work hard to prepare; then trust your preparation.

Second, surround yourself with encouraging people. It can be helpful to find a study group, but be sure that the people you're around will encourage a positive attitude. If you spend time with others who are anxious or cynical, this will only contribute to your own anxiety. Look for others who are motivated to study hard from a desire to succeed, not from a fear of failure.

Third, reward yourself. A test is physically and mentally tiring, even without anxiety, and it can be helpful to have something to look forward to. Plan an activity following the test, regardless of the outcome, such as going to a movie or getting ice cream.

When you are taking the test, if you find yourself beginning to feel anxious, remind yourself that you know the material. Visualize successfully completing the test. Then take a few deep, relaxing breaths and return to it. Work through the questions carefully but with confidence, knowing that you are capable of succeeding.

Developing a healthy mental approach to test taking will also aid in other areas of life. Test anxiety affects more than just the actual test—it can be damaging to your mental health and even contribute to depression. It's important to beat test anxiety before it becomes a problem for more than testing.

Study Strategy

Being prepared for the test is necessary to combat anxiety, but what does being prepared look like? You may study for hours on end and still not feel prepared. What you need is a strategy for test prep. The next few pages outline our recommended steps to help you plan out and conquer the challenge of preparation.

Step 1: Scope Out the Test

Learn everything you can about the format (multiple choice, essay, etc.) and what will be on the test. Gather any study materials, course outlines, or sample exams that may be available. Not only will this help you to prepare, but knowing what to expect can help to alleviate test anxiety.

Step 2: Map Out the Material

Look through the textbook or study guide and make note of how many chapters or sections it has. Then divide these over the time you have. For example, if a book has 15 chapters and you have five days to study, you need to cover three chapters each day. Even better, if you have the time, leave an extra day at the end for overall review after you have gone through the material in depth.

If time is limited, you may need to prioritize the material. Look through it and make note of which sections you think you already have a good grasp on, and which need review. While you are studying, skim quickly through the familiar sections and take more time on the challenging parts.

Write out your plan so you don't get lost as you go. Having a written plan also helps you feel more in control of the study, so anxiety is less likely to arise from feeling overwhelmed at the amount to cover.

Step 3: Gather Your Tools

Decide what study method works best for you. Do you prefer to highlight in the book as you study and then go back over the highlighted portions? Or do you type out notes of the important information? Or is it helpful to make flashcards that you can carry with you? Assemble the pens, index cards, highlighters, post-it notes, and any other materials you may need so you won't be distracted by getting up to find things while you study.

If you're having a hard time retaining the information or organizing your notes, experiment with different methods. For example, try color-coding by subject with colored pens, highlighters, or post-it notes. If you learn better by hearing, try recording yourself reading your notes so you can listen while in the car, working out, or simply sitting at your desk. Ask a friend to quiz you from your flashcards, or try teaching someone the material to solidify it in your mind.

Step 4: Create Your Environment

It's important to avoid distractions while you study. This includes both the obvious distractions like visitors and the subtle distractions like an uncomfortable chair (or a too-comfortable couch that makes you want to fall asleep). Set up the best study environment possible: good lighting and a comfortable work area. If background music helps you focus, you may want to turn it on, but otherwise keep the room quiet. If you are using a computer to take notes, be sure you don't have any other windows open, especially applications like social media, games, or anything else that could distract you. Silence your phone and turn off notifications. Be sure to keep water close by so you stay hydrated while you study (but avoid unhealthy drinks and snacks).

Also, take into account the best time of day to study. Are you freshest first thing in the morning? Try to set aside some time then to work through the material. Is your mind clearer in the afternoon or evening? Schedule your study session then. Another method is to study at the same time of day that you will take the test, so that your brain gets used to working on the material at that time and will be ready to focus at test time.

Step 5: Study!

Once you have done all the study preparation, it's time to settle into the actual studying. Sit down, take a few moments to settle your mind so you can focus, and begin to follow your study plan. Don't give in to distractions or let yourself procrastinate. This is your time to prepare so you'll be ready to fearlessly approach the test. Make the most of the time and stay focused.

Of course, you don't want to burn out. If you study too long you may find that you're not retaining the information very well. Take regular study breaks. For example, taking five minutes out of every hour to walk briskly, breathing deeply and swinging your arms, can help your mind stay fresh.

As you get to the end of each chapter or section, it's a good idea to do a quick review. Remind yourself of what you learned and work on any difficult parts. When you feel that you've mastered the material, move on to the next part. At the end of your study session, briefly skim through your notes again.

But while review is helpful, cramming last minute is NOT. If at all possible, work ahead so that you won't need to fit all your study into the last day. Cramming overloads your brain with more information than it can process and retain, and your tired mind may struggle to recall even previously learned information when it is overwhelmed with last-minute study. Also, the urgent nature of cramming and the stress placed on your brain contribute to anxiety. You'll be more likely to go to the test feeling unprepared and having trouble thinking clearly.

So don't cram, and don't stay up late before the test, even just to review your notes at a leisurely pace. Your brain needs rest more than it needs to go over the information again. In fact, plan to finish your studies by noon or early afternoon the day before the test. Give your brain the rest of the day to relax or focus on other things, and get a good night's sleep. Then you will be fresh for the test and better able to recall what you've studied.

Step 6: Take a Practice Test

Many courses offer sample tests, either online or in the study materials. This is an excellent resource to check whether you have mastered the material, as well as to prepare for the test format and environment.

Check the test format ahead of time: the number of questions, the type (multiple choice, free response, etc.), and the time limit. Then create a plan for working through them. For example, if you have 30 minutes to take a 60-question test, your limit is 30 seconds per question. Spend less time on the questions you know well so that you can take more time on the difficult ones.

If you have time to take several practice tests, take the first one open book, with no time limit. Work through the questions at your own pace and make sure you fully understand them. Gradually work up to taking a test under test conditions: sit at a desk with all study materials put away and set a timer. Pace yourself to make sure you finish the test with time to spare and go back to check your answers if you have time.

After each test, check your answers. On the questions you missed, be sure you understand why you missed them. Did you misread the question (tests can use tricky wording)? Did you forget the information? Or was it something you hadn't learned? Go back and study any shaky areas that the practice tests reveal.

Taking these tests not only helps with your grade, but also aids in combating test anxiety. If you're already used to the test conditions, you're less likely to worry about it, and working through tests until you're scoring well gives you a confidence boost. Go through the practice tests until you feel comfortable, and then you can go into the test knowing that you're ready for it.

Test Tips

On test day, you should be confident, knowing that you've prepared well and are ready to answer the questions. But aside from preparation, there are several test day strategies you can employ to maximize your performance.

First, as stated before, get a good night's sleep the night before the test (and for several nights before that, if possible). Go into the test with a fresh, alert mind rather than staying up late to study.

Try not to change too much about your normal routine on the day of the test. It's important to eat a nutritious breakfast, but if you normally don't eat breakfast at all, consider eating just a protein bar. If you're a coffee drinker, go ahead and have your normal coffee. Just make sure you time it so that the caffeine doesn't wear off right in the middle of your test. Avoid sugary beverages, and drink enough water to stay hydrated but not so much that you need a restroom break 10 minutes into the test. If your test isn't first thing in the morning, consider going for a walk or doing a light workout before the test to get your blood flowing.

Allow yourself enough time to get ready, and leave for the test with plenty of time to spare so you won't have the anxiety of scrambling to arrive in time. Another reason to be early is to select a good seat. It's helpful to sit away from doors and windows, which can be distracting. Find a good seat, get out your supplies, and settle your mind before the test begins.

When the test begins, start by going over the instructions carefully, even if you already know what to expect. Make sure you avoid any careless mistakes by following the directions.

Then begin working through the questions, pacing yourself as you've practiced. If you're not sure on an answer, don't spend too much time on it, and don't let it shake your confidence. Either skip it and come back later, or eliminate as many wrong answers as possible and guess among the remaining ones. Don't dwell on these questions as you continue—put them out of your mind and focus on what lies ahead.

Be sure to read all of the answer choices, even if you're sure the first one is the right answer. Sometimes you'll find a better one if you keep reading. But don't second-guess yourself if you do immediately know the answer. Your gut instinct is usually right. Don't let test anxiety rob you of the information you know.

If you have time at the end of the test (and if the test format allows), go back and review your answers. Be cautious about changing any, since your first instinct tends to be correct, but make sure you didn't misread any of the questions or accidentally mark the wrong answer choice. Look over any you skipped and make an educated guess.

At the end, leave the test feeling confident. You've done your best, so don't waste time worrying about your performance or wishing you could change anything. Instead, celebrate the successful completion of this test. And finally, use this test to learn how to deal with anxiety even better next time.

Review Video: Test Anxiety
Visit mometrix.com/academy and enter code: 100340

Important Qualification

Not all anxiety is created equal. If your test anxiety is causing major issues in your life beyond the classroom or testing center, or if you are experiencing troubling physical symptoms related to your anxiety, it may be a sign of a serious physiological or psychological condition. If this sounds like your situation, we strongly encourage you to seek professional help.

Online Resources

Due to our efforts to try to keep this book to a manageable length, we've created a link that will give you access to all of your online resources:

mometrix.com/resources719/oncnutrition

It's Your Moment, Let's Celebrate It!

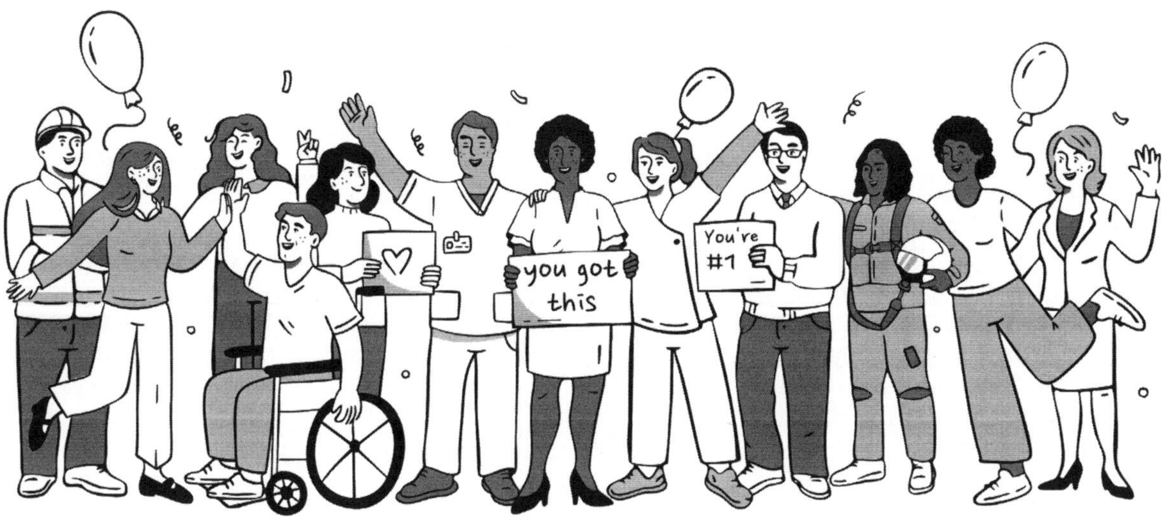

Share your story @mometrixtestpreparation